THE ART OF TRIAGE

Nursing – Issues, Problems and Challenges

Additional books in this series can be found on Nova's website under the Series tab.

Additional e-books in this series can be found on Nova's website under the e-book tab.

NURSING - ISSUES, PROBLEMS AND CHALLENGES

THE ART OF TRIAGE

TRACY ANNE EDWARDS

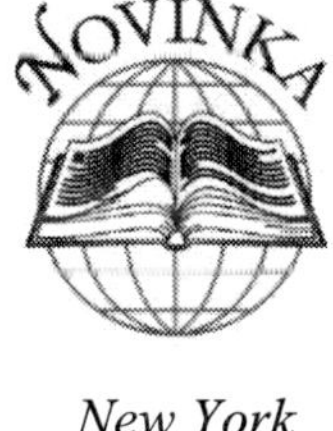

NOVINKA

New York

Library of Congress Cataloging-in-Publication Data

ISBN: 978-1-62808-592-1
LCCN: 2013944997

Published by Nova Science Publishers, Inc.† New York

To my wonderful husband Paul who has shown nothing but support for me during my nursing career. To my fantastic daughters Jessica and Laura, who have helped give me time to write this book, to my wonderful colleagues Kathryn, Michelle and Lecia my proof reader, I could not have done this without your support and guidance, and finally Lynda and the staff at Modbury Hospital Emergency Department who have supported me in my journey to becoming a Nurse Practitioner.

CONTENTS

PREFACE

This book has been written for nurses, it contains information regarding the history of triage and the different triage systems used throughout the world. I have written this book to assist nurses in understanding the reasoning behind triage and the importance of categorising patients according to the severity of illness. This book also has triage scenarios that are designed to encourage the beginning triage nurse to think about the process of triage and the types of questions they can ask the patient to ascertain a correct triage category or score. The scenarios are provided for nurses to gain confidence in the triage process.

This book also looks at critical thinking / reasoning as this is an important part of the triage process. Nurses use critical thinking every day in the care they provide their patients but at triage they use this vital skill to assess and provide a triage score to patients presenting who can potentially be critically ill. The triage nurses role is vital in ensuring patients receive the correct triage score according to the acuity of their condition. Critical thinking plays an significant role here as nurses rely on being able to problem solve, prioritise and synthesise information provided by the patient culminating in a triage score being allocated to that particular patient. This book touches on why critical thinking is important.

Tracy Edwards, RN
Emergency Nurse Practitioner
Modbury Hospital Emergency Department
Modbury, Adelaide South Australia
tracy.edwards@health.sa.gov.au

Chapter 1

HISTORY OF TRIAGE

ABSTRACT

This chapter steps the reader through the history of triage since its inception during the Napoleonic Wars in the 1800's to today's civilian form of triage. Triage in its early form was used by Baron Dominique Jean Larrey and was used in many world wars and conflicts since then. Triage was initially used in the military form, today it is used in civilian emergency departments [ED] as a way of prioritising patients in regards to their urgency of care.

INTRODUCTION

This chapter describes the history of triage and how the system used to assess patients clinical urgency [1]. Triage has been used to assess patients since the Napoleonic Wars in the 18th century. The origin of the word triage "trier" is French and means to "separate out", another definition is "the assignment of degrees of urgency to wounds or illnesses to decide the order of treatment of a large number of patients or casualties" [1]. Triage is a system used to assess the acuity of patient's as they present to the [ED].

DOMINIQUE JEAN LARREY (1766-1844) / NAPOLEONIC WARS

When talking about triage one must look back to the 1700s, Napoleon Bonaparte (1769-1821) and the Napoleonic Wars 18th century where triage was first used to assess injured soldiers in battle. Baron Dominique Jean Larrey (1766-1842), was a battlefield surgeon and during the Italy campaign, won the admiration of Napoleon Bonaparte and spent 18 years in Napoleon's imperial guard throughout the Napoleonic Wars. He accompanied Napoleon on 25 campaigns, 60 battles and more than 400 engagements [1].

Larrey has been described as the father of modern military surgery [1]. Larrey started his career as a naval surgeon, but suffered sea sickness; so decided to give up his career as a naval surgeon, transferring to the army he became an army surgeon honing in on his skills as a battlefield surgeon. It was during this time when Larrey realised the many difficulties on the battlefield. He could see the problems experienced by the wounded, and the difficulties retrieving the wounded and providing them with effective care. Wounded were not seen as a priority for the advancing army, so many of the wounded would remain on the battlefield usually until the end of the engagement; this meant that they lay dying on the battlefield for 24 hours and often died[1].

Barron Larrey was revolutionary in his ideas for the removal of wounded soldiers from the battlefield. Barron Larrey developed the flying ambulances, or ambulance volantes, as he called them; which were light horse drawn ambulances that were used for rapid evacuation of the wounded from the battlefields. The injured soldiers were then transferred to bigger ambulances at the rear of the battlefield. The wounded were treated in the rear of these bigger ambulances where they had dressing stations and then on to hospital. As the ambulances waited for the end of the battle to collect the wounded some soldiers went without treatment for 24-36 hours and therefore many of them died. Larrey was known for treating the injured no matter their rank or country and this is the tradition that has been carried on throughout the years by many countries it is the essence of military medicine [5].

History tells us that ambulances were used for the first time in 1796-97 campaign in Italy; when Barron Larrey was under the command of young Bonaparte. These ambulances were more than just forms of transport to remove the wounded from the battlefield; they were equipped with bandages, supplies, food and provisions to treat wounded horses [3, 4] the medical staff were really "jack of all trades" caring for humans and animals. In essence, this is where triage first began.

Barron Larrey died in 1842 a day after his beloved wife, his son Hippolyte who was also a surgeon asked that he be buried in the gardens of the military hospital Les Invalides this was his last request but it was denied, he was buried in the Pere Lachaise cemetery. On December 15th 1992 exactly 150 years after his death Larrey got his final wish and was buried at Les Invalides in a special ceremony [3].

Barron Larrey was a true humanitarian, he was dismayed to see how the wounded were treated and left to die on the battlefields and this prompted him to develop his system of the flying ambulances. Larrey was not only known for this development he was also an accomplished surgeon in his own right he saved many lives with his radical amputations which he sometimes performed at the rear of the battlefield. Larrey himself was injured during one of these campaigns but once recovered he was back on duty performing a job that he loved.

AMERICAN CIVIL WAR (1861-1865)

During the civil war in the United States of America (USA) they used an ad hoc system of triage where immediate treatment was provided for injuries such a gunshot wounds to extremities. This form of triage was known as field triage and was used on the battlefield; subsequent wars used a form of field triage as well although it evolved to also involve evacuation. Treatment provided was commonly the amputation of the affected limb, the walking wounded were left and received treatment later as they were not as severely injured. Soldiers who had sustained gunshot wounds to the abdomen were often left to die as there was a lack of resources to deal with this type of injury and there was also lack of knowledge on the part of the doctors.

Dr Jonathon Letterman was a field surgeon during the civil war and he was responsible for the initiation of a field ambulance service which removed the soldiers from the battlefield, similar to the work of Barron Jean Larrey. He also developed the staged evacuation of casualties; the first stage was removal from the battlefield to a field dressing station usually located on or very close to the battlefield. The second stage was transport to a field hospital which was located not far from the battlefield and the third stage was transport to a larger field hospital away from the battlefield [7].

This form of field triage was used in many wars and campaigns to come and was adapted and evolved as the forms of evacuation became more mechanised.

WORLD WAR I (1914-1918) / WORLD WAR II (1939-1945)

The great wars of the 20th century arrived and the triage system had improved vastly, a more formal tiered form of triage had been developed. This form of triage had advanced further from World War I and into World War II; there was further advancement by the time the Korean War commenced. In World War I they proposed that the treatment of the minor wounded should occur first as these soldiers could be returned to the battlefield [8], this continued during World War II. General Omar Bradley a World War II commander would later describe Dr Letterman's 3 stage removal of wounded soldiers from the battlefield as one of the greatest innovations in military medicine. The military has used this staged evacuation well and it is from this body of work that triage today has evolved, although civilian triage treats the seriously ill first and leaves the walking wounded to wait a little longer.

KOREAN WAR (1950-1953) / VIETNAM WAR (1962 -1975)

When the Korean War started the triage system was a 4 tier staged transport where patients where moved to higher levels of care if required, this was the first time air transport was used to evacuate patients. The time to treatment during the Korean War was now down to 2-4 hours from 12-18 hours during the Second World War [8]. Triage and removal of wounded from the battlefield had come a long way from the days of Barron Dominique Larrey in 1796, to the commencement of the Korean War in 1950. Air transport was used to remove casualties from the battlefield, in Korea, helicopters used had limited capacity to carry patients and could not fly in bad weather, this progressed in the Vietnam War where the use of helicopters continued due to the terrain and they were larger of course allowing multiple evacuations at one time [6]. The possibility of survival from the wounds sustained had increased and soldiers were receiving better care outcomes.

CIVILIAN TRIAGE

Wartime triage systems look at prioritising care to the injured and how they are going to evacuate them to facilities for higher levels of care. Civilian triage in EDs also looks at the acuity of the patient but also takes into account the time the patient can wait for the commencement of treatment and what treatment area they should be allocated. In the 1950s and 1960s triage moved from the military type triage to civilian triage. In the 1950s in the USA doctors provided surgery based health care along with home visits, this started to change and surgeries were closing in the evenings so patients had no where to go to seek medical treatment. This in turn placed increased pressure on the ED, patients presented to the ED with minor injuries and illness not requiring immediate care was becoming an issue they had to manage [2].

This form of civilian triage was first introduced in the USA at Parkland Hospital in Dallas Texas; it was the first to commence nurse initiated triage. There was opposition at the beginning about nurses not having the skill, knowledge or clinical experience to perform triage, medical staff thought it their domain [2]. In the 1970s and 1980s Canada were looking at triage and were looking at implementing the American system, in England they implemented an experimental triage system in Nottinghamshire in an attempt to reduce wait times and determine patient opinion.

In the 1990s enough research had been done to show that waiting times had been reduced so hospitals around the world started to look at what was the best system for them. In 1998 two ED physicians from the USA Dr Richard Wuerz and Dr David Eitel developed the Emergency Severity Index (ESI). At the same time (ED)s around the world were also researching triage methods, in 1993 in Australia the National Triage Scale was introduced and this evolved into the Australian Triage Scale (ATS) which is used today.

The Canadian triage scale was developed in 1997 and is named the Canadian Triage and Acuity Scale (CTAS) and has been in use since this time. The Manchester Triage Scale (MTS) was developed by the Manchester Triage Group which was composed of a group of ED physicians and nurses and commenced operation in 1994 this system has also been adopted by some European countries.

All of these triage systems used throughout the world have been widely researched and have gone through many revisions and updates to ensure they are valid and provide the best care for the patients presenting to (ED) s. The triage systems have also had the input of emergency physicians and nurses who have spent many hours researching and developing the systems that we use today.

Triage both military and civilian has come a long way since the times of Baron Larrey in the 1800's although the need to prioritise care has not changed. Patients presenting to (ED) s must be prioritised according to the acuity of their condition to ensure the sickest are treated first.

REFERENCES

[1]   Skandalakis. P, Panagiotis.L, Odyseas Z, et al. (2006) "To Afford the Wounded Speedy Assistance": Dominique Jean Larrey and Napoleon. *World Journal of Surgery*, 2006. (30), pp 1392-1399

[2]   Lahdet. Eric. (2009) Analysis of triage worldwide, *Emergency Nurse*. July 2009. Vol 17, No4

[3]   Welling. David, Burris. David, Rich. Norman. (2006) Delayed Recognition – Larrey and Les Invalides. *Journal American College of Surgeons*, Vol 202, No 2, February 2006, pp 373-376

[4]   DiGioia. Julie, Rocko. Joyce, Swan. Kenneth. (1983) Barron Larrey, Modern Military Surgeon, *The American Surgeon*, Vol 49, No 5, May 1983, pp 226-239

[5]   Burris. David, Welling. David, Rich, Norman. (2004) Dominique Jean Larrey and the Principles of Humanity in Warfare. *Journal American College of Surgeons*, Vol 198, No 5, May 2004, pp 831-835

[6]   Kelly. Patrick (2003) Vietnam, 1968-1969: A Place and a Year Like No Other. *Neurosurgery*, Vol 52, No 4, April 2003 pp 927-943

[7]   Greenwood, John T. (2003). Hammond and Letterman: A tale of two men who changed army medicine. *Landpower Essay,* No 03-1. June 2003, downloaded from http://www.ausa.org/SiteCollectionDocuments/ILW%20Web-ExclusivePubs/Landpower%20Essays/LPE03-1.pdf. January 2013

[8]   Iserson. Kenneth V, Moskop. John C (2007) Triage in Medicine, Part I: Concept, History, and Types. *Annals of Emergency Medicine,* Vol 49, No3, March 2007, pp 275-287 downloaded February 2013 from http://instructor.mstc.edu/instructor/randers/documents/Triage%20in%20Medicine.pdf

Chapter 2

TRIAGE SYSTEMS

ABSTRACT

This chapter will outline what triage is, why it is an integral part of the smooth running of the (ED) and what systems are used throughout the world. There are many different triage systems that are available worldwide today; at present there are many systems in use to assess the urgency of care required by patients who present to (ED) s. This chapter explains the triage systems used, in Australia, Canada, USA, and the United Kingdom (UK) from the authors perspective.

The author works within the Australian triage system and has 29 years nursing experience with 10 years of emergency nursing experience. Triage requires experience as a nurse, a sound knowledge base, excellent critical thinking skills to perform the role of triage nurse effectively, this chapter explains the role of triage and how triage is used to prioritise care.

INTRODUCTION

When patients present to any (ED) around the world they are subject to a process called triage. This process allows the ED nurse to assess, formulate a quick nursing diagnosis, allocate a category of urgency and then move the patients to the correct treatment areas. It is this category of urgency that is allocated to the patient that decides how quickly they are to have treatment commenced. There are many forms of triage used throughout the world, not all countries use the same triage scoring systems.

In the United Kingdom, Ireland and some European countries they use the Manchester Triage System (MTS). In Canada they use the Canadian Triage and Acuity Scale (CTAS), the United States of America use the Emergency Severity Index (ESI) and in Australia and New Zealand we use the Australasian Triage Scale (ATS).

The different triage scales and scoring systems one uses to assess patients as they present to the ED, all have the same outcome. Patients are given a category / priority which correlates to a time that treatment should commence.

TRIAGE, WHAT IS IT?

Triage is the process for determining the priority of patients treatment based on the severity of their condition [1], triage is a complex decision making process [4]. The term comes from the French verb "trier" which means to separate, sift or select [2]. Triage has been used since the time of Baron Larrey who used a form of triage during the Napoleonic Wars. Since then triage has evolved, in the 1950's and 1960's triage evolved from the military form to the civilian triage we use today [3]. The reason for the transformation was due to the fact that doctor's surgeries were closed after hours and on weekends patients presented to (ED) s.

As more patients presented to (ED) s this placed extra stress on these departments. The (ED) had to come up with a way of prioritising care for these patients. When civilian triage was introduced doctors initially performed this role. They performed triage and determined patients need for care. In 1962, Parkland Hospital in Dallas Texas became the first hospital to use a nurse to perform this role. Parkland became a model for other hospitals across the Unites States [3].

There has always been opposition to nurses performing triage. Initially medical staff felt that nurses lacked the expertise or clinical knowledge to perform this vital ED role. Triage today is used worldwide in (ED) s. A rating scale / score is necessary to ensure that the right order of treatment is followed, especially when there is high demand in the ED [4]. This ensures the safety and quality of care provided to patients presenting to the ED.

Farrohknia (2011) states "triage scales aim to optimise the waiting time of patients according to the severity of their medical condition, in order to treat as fast as necessary the most intense symptom(s) and to reduce the negative impact on the prognosis of a prolonged delay before treatment" pg 1. The process of triage is completed to determine a patient's acuity level [5]. A patient's acuity level is defined as the urgency for effective care (Towmey 2012). Towmey 2012 states "In the ED triage setting effective care is defined as the provision of an intervention or treatment that reduces the patient's urgency for care or presents clinical deterioration" pg 477.

In this instance the triage nurse can commence some form of treatment for the patient while they await assessment by the physician. It may be the administration of pain relief, applying ice to a suspected fracture / sprain or elevation of a painful leg. All of these treatments can alleviate the patient suffering while they wait to be seen according to their acuity assigned by the triage nurse.

If patients receive timely and effective care, triage has achieved its purpose. It is important that the triage process has validity and reliability. This means that it is important that the same assessment of a patient will deliver the same acuity level. It also means that the degree of acuity assessed actually reflects the acuity of the patient at the time of triage [5]. It must be noted that effective triage uses not only sight but hearing, smell and touch as well [13]. The triage nurse listens to what patients say they may hear them cough which will give them information, they may feel the pulse or smell ketones or alcohol. All of this information aids in their triage allocation [13], and demonstrates the nurse showing empathy and caring as to why the patient has presented to the ED.

When the nurse assesses the patient and makes a triage decision they rely on both subjective and objective data obtained from the patient to make a decision as to what category / priority to assign that patient. The nurse asks the patient questions about the reason for presentation to elicit information that will enable them to make an accurate assessment of the patient. While they are talking to the patient the nurse is also observing the patient, they may take some quick vital signs or pulse oximetry, they may ascertain a pain score [3].

It is after this questioning of the patient and observing their condition, and / or vital signs the nurse will give the patient a triage category / priority. This priority decides how quickly the patient requires care. It is this rating that indicates how long the patient is able to wait for the commencement of care [6]. If the patient is unable to answer any questions, obtaining information from a third party, accompanying person or significant other is important. Information obtained about the presenting complaint and past medical history can assist the nurse in allocating a triage priority / category. There are many reasons why a patient may not be able to answer the triage nurses questions, these can range from intellectual disability, deaf or mute patients, the elderly and those in acute pain are just a few examples. The triage nurse must obtain information for other sources to enable them to make the correct decision for this particular presentation.

There are many factors that nurses must be aware of when patients present to the triage counter. The physical environment of the triage area can play an important part in the ability of the triage nurse to communicate effectively with the patient. Many departments have triage areas with desks, bullet proof glass and a lack of privacy. Patients present to the triage desk and speak to the nurse through these barriers. It is the skill of the triage nurse that can overcome these barriers with good communication.

Patients present to the triage nurse with sometimes very private and embarrassing illnesses and injuries. The skill of the triage nurse is vital, it is their role to question the patient and determine the nature of the illness ensuring the patient does not suffer any embarrassment. As triage nurses we must remember that patients present to the triage desk with pre conceptions and assumptions of what is going to occur. They feel unwell or are injured and they want to be treated immediately. The triage nurse is the first person they meet so it is part of their role to ensure patients understand what to expect once they have registered. There have been studies done in the past looking at whether it makes the patients journey easier if they are informed of what their triage category is and how long they will have to wait for treatment to commence [13].

In some emergency departments they do display an up to date waiting time so that patients are kept informed. The department where the author works does not display a wait time, when patients are triaged they are informed they may have either a short or long wait. They are informed that the department has two streams one called fast track where the priority four and five patients are seen and the other stream for the patient who requires a cubicle and more in depth care.

The triage nurse should be able to make an assessment of the patient's condition within 3-5 minutes of questioning them. It is important to take into account verbal and non-verbal language of the patient. Not using medical jargon is also important; patients do not understand the medical jargon that we as medical and nursing professionals use. It is important to use clear language that the patient can understand such as not asking the patient if they have "abdominal" pain but asking them if they have "tummy" or "stomach" pain. The triage nurse should be able to judge who can understand certain types of language, as the last thing they want to do is to offend the patient by treating them like a child.

The non verbal language of the triage nurse is also important, the tone of the triage nurses questioning, their body language, facial expressions and posture are all aspects of communication. Patients will pick up on these cues and depending will provide the nurse with enough information to make a clinical decision what triage category / priority to allocate the patient.

egory 1- Immediately Life Threatening / Immediate

Patients allocated the category 1 level do not always present to the (ED) via ambulance service they can still present as a walk in patient. Many cardiac ents will present as walk ins for reasons only known to them they do not call ambulance. Patients in the category 1 level require treatment urgently and mediately.

Look at the asthma presentation in the category 2, this type of patient can ite easily be allocated a priority 1. If the patient had presented to the triage desk t able to breath with an airway that was more obstructed or compromised the iage nurse could quite easily justify allocating this patient a priority 1. The atient that presents to the triage desk with severe chest pain, that looks pale and iaphoretic that collapses in front of the desk is quite clearly a priority 1.

These types of presentations can occur as the patient may not have ambulance cover and are too worried over the cost to call an ambulance. They may not realise just how unwell they actually are and feel the drive to the hospital is OK, and finally they may have deteriorated on their way to the hospital. There are many reasons why patients present as a walk in and not via the ambulance service and they can be provided education about the importance of calling an ambulance at a later date, educating patients during a stressful situation is not appropriate and they may not take in all the information provided.

Patients that may present in this category include cardiac or respiratory arrest, major trauma, major haemorrhage, airway obstruction especially in children and the fitting patient.

Category 2- Imminently Life Threatening /10 Minutes

A patient presenting to the triage window stating they are short of breath and they are having an asthma attack is a different story. The triage nurse in this situation would have some information already from visually looking at the patient, they may appear short of breath, they may have a wheeze the nurse can hear which should ring alarm bells in regards to an airway obstruction, and they

on how the nurse presents themselves communication could become difficult. Communication is vital in the triage process, the triage nurses body language and how they engage the patient is important. How patients perceive the triage nurses body language may play a role in the patient feeling at ease enough to provide accurate information.

The emotional side of triage is another important factor to consider. Nurses react to stressful situations in all different ways and so do patients. It is important from the triage nurses perspective that they remain calm and keep an even tone, neutral body language and do not become emotional. Patients also can become emotional when telling their stories; this can lead to miss information and an inability to provide coherent / useful information. Another factor that must be considered is that of cultural diversity, an elderly man presenting to triage may not want to explain their condition to a young woman. This must be taken into account, also patients from different cultures must also be respected and when possible allowances made to make the patient feel comfortable.

Triage nurses must ensure that that they are not judgemental or prejudiced when listening to the patient explain why they have presented as this can lead to moral judgements and then mistakes are also made. If the triage nurse judges the patient they are at risk of allocating the wrong triage category / priority and this can lead to adverse outcomes for the patient.

Before triage scales were introduced many (ED) s saw patients in order of arrival, like many of the after hour's medical surgeries. In Australia there are after hours medical surgeries that do not require a patient to have an appointment, the patients are seen in order of arrival time. Since 1990 many countries developed and introduced triage scales, several countries developed the 5 tier triage scales. Of these triage scales there are four that have had the greatest influence on modern triage practices in (ED)s, and they are listed below;

1. Australasian Triage Scale (ATS)
2. Canadian (ED) Triage and Acuity Scale (CTAS)
3. Manchester Triage Scale (MTS) and the
4. Emergency Severity Index (ESI)

Other triage scales such as the Soterion Rapid Triage Scale (SRTS) from the United States and the four tier Taiwan Triage System (TTS) have not made such an impact worldwide. Australia uses a national triage scale where as many European countries lack such national standards [4]. In South Africa they have adapted the Medical Early Warning Score (MEWS) score and use this as a basis for their triage system. South Africa use the Emergency Triage Assessment and Treatment scale it is also used in India, Malawi and Brazil.

So let's look at the four major triage systems used throughout the world starting with the Australasian Triage Scale (ATS).

AUSTRALASIAN TRIAGE SCALE (ATS)

Australian triage was developed in the 1970s where a five tier scale was used at the Box Hill hospital in Victoria, it was refined and became the Ipswich Triage Scale in the 1980s and then was further refined to become the National Triage Scale [13]. The Australasian Triage Scale was adapted from the previous scale used called the National Triage Scale (NTS). The NTS was formally introduced into (ED) s in 1993, this was the first system used in Australian (ED) s [7].

As in all evidenced based nursing and medicine the NTS underwent review and was renamed the Australasian Triage Scale (ATS). The ATS is a 5 tier triage system, it is an acuity system used for allocating a triage score to a patient on presentation to the ED.

The ATS has a scale of 1-5 as follows;

Category 1 – Immediately life-threatening
Category 2 – Imminently life-threatening
Category 3 – Potentially life-threatening or important time-critical treatment
    or severe pain
Category 4 – potentially life-serious or situational urgency or significant
    complexity
Category 5 – Less urgent

Each of the five levels of acuity has a time for assessment and the commencement of treatment attached to them as follows [8];

Category1 – Immediate care
Category2 - within 10 minutes
Category 3 – within 30 minutes
Category 4 - within 60 minutes and
Category 5 – within 120 minutes

When the NTS was reviewed and changed to the ATS were reviewed and some inclusions were made. Category one and the category two descriptors had some inclusions add inclusions were expanded to include the patient presenting presentations such as ectopic pregnancy, those in severe pai emergencies such as violence or self-harm. The category three also reviewed and expanded to include most fractures, head injuri The category five descriptors were reduced to reflect the time pati to be seen. This category included those with very minor injuries, issues such as medical certificates, prescription and those with stable

Nurses within the Australian health system prior to taking on the generally have many years nursing and emergency nursing experie working at triage. Some nurses would have completed post graduate emergency nursing. With the ATS triage system the triage nurse has u triage learning package which was developed by the Department of Ageing which is an Australian Federal Government Department. The p named The Emergency Triage Education Kit (ETEK) and has been deve many doctors, nurses, peak education and professional bodies who worl the emergency nursing and medicine field.

The ATS system is a concise and easy triage system to use once the nu completed the appropriate training and orientation. Most (ED) s in Australi have an orientation program that they use to train and orientate nurses to the system and role. This will involve completing the ETEK package and one or day's orientation to the triage role with a senior nurse providing support education on the job this can differ from institution to institution. The ETEK case scenarios as part of the training program so the nurse can assess the patie and make the correct triage decision.

It must be remembered that there is no right or wrong answer in the triage decision made by the nurse but the decision as to what category or priority the patient is allocated can affect the care provided to that patient and whether they have a positive or negative experience or outcome. The triage nurse carries a great deal of responsibility on their shoulders to assess the patient thoroughly and make a good decision. There is nothing stopping the triage nurse from re-assessing the patient and up-triaging them if they feel the patient's condition has changed and requires treatment more urgently.

When a patient presents to the ED they are greeted by the triage nurse and asked why they have presented today, the patient may give a simple explanation may appear shaky especially if they have used their salbutamol puffer or nebuliser frequently. The nurse would already have assessed airway, breathing and circulation as the patient is standing in front of them and they have taken their pulse on arrival. The nurse may perform oxygen saturation while they are questioning the patient. The nurse will then ask some questions such as have you used your asthma medications? How many times have you used them? Do you feel they are working?

If the oxygen (O^2) saturation is low (less than 95 per cent) and the patient is unable to speak in sentences this should ring alarm bells and the triage nurse will allocate the patient a priority 2 meaning the patient must be seen within 10 minutes and treatment commenced. This type of presentation is a common occurrence in many (ED) s' around the world and can be potentially life threatening. The difficulty for the triage nurse is with this type of presentation the patient may have stayed at home and struggled to treat themselves for many hours prior to presentation to the (ED). If they can only speak in words this type of history is very difficult to obtain at triage, the nurse must rely on their visual skills and the limited information obtained from the patient to make a triage decision.

These types of patients with this presentation can deteriorate quickly and potentially have an adverse outcome, they may not require immediate care but they are not the type of patient that the nurse wants sitting in the waiting room for any length of time so a priority 2 is the right score to allocate this patient. The patient with chest pain also fits into this category and the triage nurse would question the patient closely looking at the onset, duration, radiation of pain, relieving factors and past medical history. These patients are required to be seen within 10 minutes the reasoning here is that if a myocardial infarction (MI) is the cause the patient will require transfer for primary angiogram / angioplasty if not available at the presenting hospital, this is a time critical presentation.

The early pregnant woman who presents stating she has abdominal pain, is pregnant, she may look pale and unwell or can look relatively well is a concern. The nurse must question the patient to ensure they obtain the correct information that allows them to allocate the correct triage category / score. If the patient looks unwell, has shoulder tip pain, is tachycardic the triage nurse should be concerned and allocate a triage 2 as they may suspect an ectopic pregnancy.

Patients that may be allocated a category 2 would include, chest pain, pneumothorax (unstable with respiratory compromise), patients with acute pain and a pain score 8/10 or above, asthma with respiratory compromise, ectopic pregnancy, febrile children who look flat and DKA.

Category 3 – Potentially Life- Threatening or Time Critical or Severe Pain-30 Minutes

An example of this type of patient would be a patient presenting to the triage desk saying that they have abdominal pain all over, have been experiencing the pain for the past 12 hours, they feel nauseated, cannot keep anything down and tell you they just don't feel right or may appear agitated. Again the nurse would be visually assessing the patient and have assessed the airway, breathing and circulation of the patient. They will ask the patient the reason for the presentation today; they may take the patients pulse as they are asking questions, to determine if the patient is tachycardic.

The types of questions the nurse may ask will assist them to formulate a nursing diagnosis and what triage category the patient will be allocated. The nurse may ask the patient exactly where the pain is and what type of pain they are experiencing, how long they have had the pain and have they taken any pain relief. Asking what relieves the pain or makes it worse is another important question as the pain may be intermittent, also asking if the pain is present now is important. Another question the nurse may ask is has the patient had their bowels opened recently. The nurse then may ask about the patients past medical history or what medications they are taking as this may allude to the cause of the abdominal pain.

The answers the nurse receives will determine the triage category that the patient is allocated. A patient with severe abdominal pain with a past medical history of hypertension that describes the pain as a tearing / pulling sensation that may be centrally located will be given a higher priority as the nurse may suspect an abdominal aortic aneurysm (AAA) compared to the patient with no past medical history stating the pain was located all over the abdomen that presents looking well and has not had their bowels opened for 5 days. The nurse may suspect the patient has constipation and can therefore wait longer for treatment to commence.

In this situation the nurse may allocate the patient with a suspected AAA a category 2 which means they must be seen within 10 minutes and the patient with the suspected constipation a category 3- 4 that indicates they must be seen with 30 - 60 minutes.

Patients that may present in the category might be stable asthma with O^2 saturations above 95 percent, appendicitis, renal colic, patients with pain score of between 4-7/10 and abdominal pain suspected constipation.

Category 4 – Potentially Life-Serious/Situational Urgency/Significant Complexity -60 Minutes

Patients presenting in the category 4 level of the ATS are those patients that can wait a period of time for treatment by a physician to commence. An example of this may be the patient has presented to the window and states they have tripped over the dog and injured their right wrist and they cannot move it anymore as it is painful. The nurse may ask they patient when this occurred, did they hit their head and what is their pain score from 0-10, the nurse will also look for any form of deformity and check if the are neurovascular intact. Depending on the answers the nurse can make a quick visual assessment and then allocate a triage category / priority. The category or priority is likely to be either a 4 or 5 meaning the patient can wait for 60-120 minutes respectively for treatment to commence. Allocating this score does not mean that some form of treatment will not be commenced for this patient; they may be given pain relief, a sling and could possibly be sent for an x-ray.

Patients in this category may include simple fractures, minor suturing, cold and flu like symptoms with normal vital signs.

Category 5 – Less Urgent-120 Minutes

Patients presenting in this category are the patients that can wait for treatment to commence, these patients may present with pain that they have had for prolonged periods of time. Patients wanting medical certificates for work fit into this category, also patients that have been recalled for wound reviews.

It is the patients in the triage category / priority 3-4 that prove to be difficult for some nurses to assess. These are the patients that may present with the vague symptoms of abdominal pain, urinary symptoms, colds and sore throats etc. This is where the triage nurses skills and experience are really required so they can discriminate between the patient that may look reasonably well but is actually quite sick and the patient that may look a little unwell but can wait a short period of time for the commencement of treatment. The skill and experience of the triage nurse here is vital, as many of these patients may be up-triaged for the wrong reasons and this can place patients at risk. If the nurse is up-triaging or over-triaging there is a risk that the patient who is really unwell will be missed and have an adverse outcome.

It is the patient with vague symptoms or those that have been unwell for a week or possibly months that can also prove to be a challenge at triage. Questioning the patient in this scenario can be quite difficult especially if the patient's condition / presentation has been an ongoing problem for several months. The triage nurse here must question the patient without offending them or trivialising their condition. Sometimes these patients have not seen a general practitioner about the problem and the (ED) is their first line of access to a medical professional.

In Australia triage nurses are not encouraged to triage away patients, the nurse may suspect the patient could wait to see a general practitioner but the patient must be assessed and given a triage priority and treatment. Patients may have seen their general practitioner and present with a letter especially if they suspect a surgical cause for the abdominal pain such as suspected appendicitis. The nurse would assess the patient as usual and decide if a priority 3 category is required which means the patient must be seen within 30 minutes.

The Australian Triage Scale (ATS) is very comprehensive and easy to use once the nurse has received the correct training; training includes completion of the case scenarios. Every hospital is different and they all have different policies and procedures for the training of triage nurses. Even the most highly educated and experienced triage nurse will have cases that require them to think critically about the case they have in front of them and on some occasions it is as simple as look, listen, feel and smell [7].

All triage nurses are taught to use all of their senses when they triage a patient, they may smell ketones, feel a rapid pulse that they suspect is supra ventricular tachycardia or hear the patient wheezing. The triage nurse will use this information to allocate a triage category / scale.

EMERGENCY SEVERITY INDEX (ESI)

As mentioned earlier the purpose of triage is to prioritise care and determine which patients are able to wait for care [9]. Historically (ED) s in the United States did not have a standardised triage rating scale. Since 2000 they have been using a five tier triage acuity rating scale and in 2002 the Emergency Nurses Association (ENA) and the American College of Emergency Physicians (ACEP) formed a Joint Triage Five Level Task Force, this task force reviewed the literature and made recommendations for (ED) s in the United States in regards to what triage system should be used.

The ESI was developed by two ED physicians Dr Richard Wuerz and Dr David Eitel in the United States in 1998. These two physicians developed the ESI as a way for triage nurses to determine who needs to be seen first and to consider what resources are required to move the patient towards disposition (admission, discharge or transfer) [9]. The first version of the ESI was introduced in 1999 at two university teaching hospitals. In 2000 it was revised with ED clinician input to include paediatrics and was then implemented in five more hospitals.

The hospitals chosen for the trial were a mix of non-university, teaching and community hospitals, after feedback from nurses and physicians at the trial sites it was further refined in 2001 as version 3. The ESI was revised again and is now version 4 which was released in 2005 along with training videos. In 2010 the ESI team released the web based training course after 10 years of research and development [9]. As shown earlier with the ATS the ESI has undergone many reviews and will undergo many more as evidenced based medicine and nursing evolves.

The ESI is a unique triage system when compared to the other triage systems in that it requires the nurse to anticipate the expected resources (*eg* diagnostic tests and procedures) along with the acuity of the patient. The acuity of the patient is the most important factor and these decisions are based on the patient's vital signs, the likelihood of life or organ threatening condition and high risk presentations. If the patient is not a high risk presentation and the triage nurse deems them stable the triage nurse predicts the resources required which is based on her experience to move the patient to disposition from the ED. The resource needs can range from one to two or more although the triage nurse does not estimate more than two resources [9].

There have been many benefits to the implementation of the ESI one of those is the ability to rapidly identify patients that require immediate attention. This is the focus of the ESI the quick sorting of patients in the setting of constrained resources [9]. This five tier triage has the ability to move the level 1 and 2 patients to areas for rapid evaluation and treatment leaving the lower acuity patients to wait safely for treatment to commence. The other benefit is patients that can wait to be assessed and be treated in an area such as fast track or non-urgent care area similar to some departments in Australia.

So what is the ESI? It is a five-level triage system used in the United States that categorises patients by their acuity level and their resource needs. The acuity level is determined by the stability of the patient's vital signs and the potential threat to life, limb or organs. The triage nurse also has to estimate the resources that may be required to treat a patient and this is done by using previous experiences of treating patients with similar presentations or injuries. Once the nurse has had training and orientation to the algorithm they should be able to rapidly assess and categorise the patients into one of the levels for treatment to commence.

The ESI unlike the Australian or the Canadian triage systems does not have a time to treatment by a physician allocated to the triage levels. However patients who meet the ESI Level-2 category should be assessed by a physician in an appropriate area as soon as possible. Again there is not a time frame allocated to the "as soon as possible "category. In the case of the chest pain patient who presents with a time –sensitive issue an ECG should be done and viewed by a physician within 10 minutes like the other triage systems.

The ESI can be broken down into the four decision points and 5 levels.

Decision Point A – ESI Level 1

Requires immediate life-saving intervention
With decision point A the triage nurse asks "does the patient require immediate life-saving intervention" if the answer here is yes the patient is allocated a Level 1 triage score and treatment commences immediately. If the nurse answers no then they move down to the next step of the algorithm to decision point B.

In this triage level the patient is requiring procedures such as management of their airway via manual ventilation, intubation or surgical airway. The may require inotropic medications to maintain blood pressure and cardiac output, and may require defibrillation / cardioversion or even external pacing. The may require chest tubes or significant fluid resuscitation, all of these procedures require immediate care from multiple sources including nurses, doctors, radiologists, and possibly specialists such as cardiology and respiratory physicians.

The ESI Level 1 patient always presents to the (ED) with unstable conditions and these are the patients who require care immediately or they may die. If the patient requires airway management, emergency medications or other haemodynamic intervention this is classed as immediate life-saving interventions. The clinical conditions that fall within this triage level include cardiac and respiratory arrest, severe respiratory distress, oxygen saturations less than 90 per cent, critically injured trauma patients, flaccid babies, severe tachycardia / bradycardia with hypoperfusion [9].

The ESI level 1 is equivalent to the ATS, CTAS and MTS level 1, all of these triage systems recognise the need for immediate life saving measures and these patients are triaged accordingly.

Decision Point B – ESI Level 2

High risk situation? Or confused / lethargic / disoriented? Or, severe pain or distress?

At this decision point the triage nurse must decide if the patient can wait to be seen; if the answer is no the patient is assigned a triage level 2. If the answer is yes the nurse then must use the next three questions to determine if the patient meets the ESI level 2 criteria.

1. Is this a high risk situation?

The nurse must use their experience as a triage nurse to quickly and briefly interview the patient, use their gross observation of how the patient presents and looks at triage. The nurse must decide if the patient has presented with a condition that has the potential to deteriorate or if they have symptoms that are time sensitive requiring treatment. This is the patient who has a potential threat to life, limb or organ. These patients do not require a detailed physical assessment or even a full set of vital signs to be done at triage.

An example of the types of presentation that is high risk can include active chest pain, needle stick in a health care worker, signs and symptoms of an acute stroke, ectopic pregnancy that is haemodynamically stable, patient on chemotherapy that is immunocompromised with a fever and a suicidal or homicidal patient [9]. These presentations are similar to the ATS category 2 patients who must be seen within 10 minutes except the needle stick injuries they are usually allocated an ATS 4 or 5.

2. Is the patient Confused, Lethargic or Disoriented?

This is the second question at decision point B and the reason for this question is to ascertain if the patient has new onset confusion or disorientation or even an acute change to their conscious state. It is important to remember patients that have a baseline state of confusion do not meet the level -2 criteria for example the patient with Alzheimer's disease. This can be difficult to assess if the onset is new especially if the patient does not have a diagnosis of dementia.

Some examples of the types of patients presenting in this category can include the new onset of confusion in the elderly, the 3 month old baby whose mother reports it is always sleeping and the adolescent who is confused and disoriented [9]. Patients in this category with the ATS system of triage may either be allocated a triage 2 or 3 depending on the history given at triage.

3. Is the Patient in Severe Pain or Distress?

This is the third question at decision point B, if the patient answers no the triage nurse moves onto the next step in the algorithm. If the answer is yes the nurse must use their clinical skills in observation and ask the patient their pain score on a scale of 0-10 with 0 being no pain and 10 being the worst ever experienced. If the patient reports the pain at 7/10 or greater the nurse may assign the patient an ESI level-2 this is not a requirement. It should be noted that pain is the most common reason for patients presenting to the ED and the triage nurse must use their clinical assessment and reasoning skills to allocate the appropriate ESI level.

An example of this would be a patient presenting with an ankle injury stating they have a pain score of 7/10 compared with a patient presenting with chest pain with the same pain score. The patient with the ankle would not receive an ESI level-2 as they can be treated with rest, ice, elevation and can wait to see a medical professional. The patient with chest pain would receive an ESI level-2 and will be seen quicker.

As stated earlier the triage nurse also has to rely on their observations skills when patients present to the triage counter, they must look, listen and feel. A patient presents to the triage counter with abdominal pain, they appear pale and unwell looking, diaphoretic and be experiencing nausea. The triage nurse might feel their pulse and determine they are tachycardic so from this observation, questioning and taking the patients pulse the triage nurse could assign the patient an ESI level-2.

When asking this question of the patient the triage nurse is not only asking questions but observing the patient's posture and their facial expressions as they relay their story.

Decision Point C - ESI Level 3-4-5

If the answer to the first two decision points is no, the triage nurse moves to the decision point C. At decision point C, the triage nurse asks how many different resources the patient requires to reach a disposition decision, which as mentioned before is admission, discharge or transfer. This decision point asks the nurse to draw on previous experience in regards to the types of presentation. The triage nurse will obtain information from the brief interview, past medical history, current medications and the presenting complaint. They will then identify the resource needs of the patient based on previous experience in the same type of presentations.

What is considered a resource? Its things like hospital services, tests, procedures, consults or interventions, all of these are above the physician history and the physical examination. An example of what is considered a resource is as follows CT, MRI or ultrasound scans, blood tests, intravenous or intramuscular medications and intravenous fluids. What is not considered a resource? The history and physical examination, point of care testing, saline or heparinized lock, immunisations or oral medications and simple wound care are all examples of what is not considered a resource.

After the triage nurse has determined how many resources the patient requires they will allocate the patient to and ESI Level, if the patient requires many resources they are allocated an ESI Level-3, if they require one resource they may be a level-4 and none a level-5.

Decision Point D – ESI Level-3

Prior to the nurse allocating an ESI Level-3 the triage nurse must look at the patient's vital signs and determine if they are outside of the accepted parameters for age. The triage nurse must make a decision here as to whether the patient should be upgraded to the ESI Level-2 category. In children under the age of 3 years the temperature is also taken into account. If the child has a significant fever this will exclude them from the category 4 and 5. The nurse must also when assessing the patient take into account the patient history given by the patient, significant other or the parents.

After working through the decision points the triage nurse allocates a triage level from 1-5 these are explained below.

Emergency Severity Index (ESI) Level-1

This level of the ESI is quite self explanatory as these are the multi trauma, cardiac and respiratory arrest, compromised airway and unconscious patients. These are the patients who will die if they do not receive life-saving treatment immediately. This is the easiest triage category to assign as the triage nurse has to ask themselves one question "will the patient die without life-saving" treatment if the answer is yes then the patient is allocated and ESI Level-1.

As mentioned earlier all of the triage systems mentioned in this book have a category or level 1 which means the patient can not wait for treatment to commence. Treatment must commence immediately, these are the patients that may die without life saving interventions.

Emergency Severity Index (ESI) Level-2

Orientating triage nurses to the ESI a considerable amount of time should be spent orientating them to the Level-2 criteria. The Level-2 criterion is important as this is the area that both under and over triage can occur. It is important to note that this is not just the case with the ESI but can also occur with other triage systems. (ED)s around the world are frequently overcrowded and the ESI Level-2 category is a category that nurses frequently struggle with especially when there are limited beds in an often busy department.

Nurses have to listen to the patient's story, visually assess the patient and make a decision as to what category to allocate this patient. The triage nurse is usually aware of the bed state in the department and they are aware of the beds available when they are allocating triage categories. When they are considering a triage Level-2 nurses need to ask themselves "would I allocate this patient the last bed in the department" or "do I ask the coordinator to move someone to make a bed for this patient" [9]. The triage nurse is required to formulate a nursing diagnosis based on the patients signs and symptoms and patient history of presenting complaint, they will also use their experience from previous presentations of this kind.

Patients that can be allocated this category include suspected AAA, chest pain, foreign body airway such as epiglottitis or oesophageal foreign body, inhalation injuries, Diabetic Ketoacidosis (DKA), sepsis, syncope, symptoms suggestive of CVA or seizure, pregnant patients with suspected ectopic pregnancy, testicular torsion, chemical splashes to the eyes, asthma and paediatric presentations such as sepsis, dehydration, febrile, ingestions, seizures, DKA, sickle cell crisis. These are just some examples of the ESI Level-2 presentation.

Emergency Severity Index (ESI)-Level 3

The two medical staff who designed the ESI believed that a triage nurse who is experienced in the ED field would be able to predict the nature and number of tests, interventions and consultations a patient would require when they present with a defined set of signs and symptoms [9]. It is at decision point C that the nurse assigns ESI levels 3-5 and the nurse is required to not only assess acuity of the patient but also the resources required to reach disposition of the patient.

The ESI levels 3, 4 and 5 are determined by the nurse assessing the patient and determining the resources required, in the ESI level-3 the patient is requiring two or more resources. So the nurse as well as taking a brief history determines if the patient requires the extra resources to reach a disposition decision. So what is considered by the nurse to be a resource? After the history the triage nurse must decide if the patient requires laboratory testing, ECG's, CT / MRI, intravenous (IV) / intramuscular (IM) or nebulised medications, specialty consultations or procedures. If the patient requires two or more of these resources they are allocated an ESI level-3.

Laboratory testing is not every single test counted as a resource, the patient may have multiple tests ordered and this is counted as one resource. If the patient is sent to radiology department and has a cervical spine x-rays and a CT of the head this is classed as two resources. Not every intervention is classed as a resource, providing the patient with ice or a simple dressing, a sling for a suspected fracture or oral pain relief are not seen as resources when triaging with the ESI system.

The reason for this is a patient with a sprained ankle for example may receive ice, oral pain relief and a wheelchair, if these were classed as a resource the patient would receive an ESI level 3 for something that is relatively minor. Examples of patients that might receive an ESI level 3could be; abdominal pain that requires laboratory testing, abdominal ultrasound, IV fluids and pain relief, the patient has required 2 or more resources or the patient that has just arrived back from a long distance flight and is complaining of left leg calf pain, they will require laboratory testing, doppler ultrasound of the leg and possibly anticoagulant therapy, this patient requires two or more resources.

The nurse must be accurate in their assessment of what resources are required for the patient when they assign the triage level as their decisions determine the patient's length of stay in the department and can impact on the patient's outcomes. In the department where the author works there is a rapid assessment team that begins treatment for this cohort of patients. Treatment may be pathology or radiology testing and a quick physician assessment.

Emergency Severity Index (ESI)-Level 4

The ESI level 4 category is an easy one as patients allocated to this category require one resource; the nurse may take the patient history and decide that the patient requires an x-ray for a sprained ankle. This is classed as one resource so the patient is allocated an ESI level 4. Patient presentations that may be allocated this category can be those with simple or minor illness like a patient with a suspected UTI, they require and urine test for MC&S and possible antibiotics. These are the types of patients that meet the ESI level 4 category.

Emergency Severity Index (ESI)-Level 5

The patients in the ESI level 5 category require no resources; these are the relatively well patients that may not be able to see their general practitioner. Some patients that may present in this category include patients that may require prescriptions if they have run out of their usual medications or the child with poison ivy (a skin irritation caused by a plant in the USA) that needs a quick examination and a prescription [9]. Both of these examples require no resources to be used beyond a simple examination of the patient. In that system most emergency departments have nurse practitioners that work within the last two categories the 4 and 5, and they are classed as the "see and treat" patients.

Looking at the ESI it could be said that it is a difficult system to use, on the other hand after reading the resources it appears the triage nurse when they are assessing the patient and asking the patient questions they are also determining what resources they may require for the patient. This is the ESI in a nutshell, it is quite a comprehensive way to triage patients as they present to the ED. The nurse assesses the patient's presenting condition and at the same time they estimate the required resources to reach dispositions then they allocate a triage level. It is a complicated system and would require an experienced triage nurse and the appropriate education to understand how to use the ESI correctly.

I have just touched on what I see as the major points of the ESI, for further information the reader can access the ESI website at www.esitriage.org , where they will find the implementation handbook and articles written describing use of the ESI. This system of triage would require the triage nurse to have many years of ED nursing experience and would require a lengthy training package and as mentioned earlier there is now a web based training packages for nurses to complete.

MANCHESTER TRIAGE SCALE (MTS)

Triage is not only a patient flow system it is also a way of managing clinical risk in the (ED). Triage allocates patients a triage level according to their clinical need and in a timely manner [9]. The Manchester Triage Group (MTS) is a group made up of senior emergency physicians and emergency nurses who came together with the aim to form a consensus about triage standards [9]. The group defined aims and these were the development of common definitions, a robust triage methodology, training package, and development of an audit guide [9].

It was found that there were considerable differences in the definitions and the times allocated for the commencement of treatment by a physician. The group has allocated a triage level, name, and colour and a maximum time to treatment in minutes; they are as follows.

Level 1 – Immediate, colour Red and 0 minutes
Level 2 – Very Urgent, colour Orange and 10 minutes
Level 3 – Urgent, colour Yellow and 60 minutes
Level 4 – Standard, colour Green and 120 minutes
Level 5 - Non-urgent, colour Blue and 240 minutes

The triage nurse attends a course which educates them on this triage system which equips them with the knowledge on how to use the triage system but not necessarily the experience. The nurse has the basics and then develops skills in using the method and the materials available to them. This system assesses patients in regards to their clinical priority by looking at their signs and symptoms, or discriminators and these discriminators are set out in flow charts.

These flow charts are called presentational flow charts. There are 50 presentational charts and two major incident charts that the triage nurse has to choose from depending on the discriminators that the patient presents to triage with. It would be too difficult to include all 50 presentational charts in this book if the reader wants more information the Manchester Triage Group has published a book which is very concise and explains the system well. The book is called "Emergency Triage" and it contains the 50 presentational flow charts and would be a great resource for any triage nurse.

This system is designed around clinical practice and the patients presenting complaint meaning the signs and symptom(s) that the patient describes on presentation to triage. The MTS group developed a list of presenting conditions after many discussions which cover the most common presentations to the ED. The group has recognised that some patients present with symptoms that may fall into more than one of the presentational charts.

The triage nurse must gather information that will enable them to allocate a triage category and to enable this they use discriminators. Discriminators can be general or specific; a general discriminator for example is severe pain while a specific one is cardiac pain [9]. The triage nurse has access to a discriminator dictionary which explains all the discriminators in the presentational flow charts. There are six general discriminators and they are life threat, haemorrhage, pain, conscious level, temperature, and acuteness [9].

Looking at the general discriminators;

Life Threat

Any compromise in airway, breathing or circulation places the patient in the level 1 / red category. These patients may present to the ED with difficulty breathing and have an audible stridor, inspiratory or expiratory wheeze which means their airway is compromised. Patients might exhibit an increased effort in breathing but show signs of inadequate oxygenation, they possibly will show signs of shock such as pallor, tachycardia, appear diaphoretic, hypotensive and may appear confused [9]. All of these conditions meet the level 1 / red category, which is the same category in the ESI, CTAS or ATS triage systems.

Pain

It must be remembered that pain is one of the main reasons patients come to the ED for treatment. It should be a major factor for determining the patient's priority and should be a question asked of all patients presenting to the ED. A recognised pain scale should be used for both adults and children; the MTS uses the pain ladders [9], page 25. This pain scale has both written and visual cues and for children has the panda faces. No one particular pain scale is better than another but a validated pain scale is important. Assessing patient's pain is important as the key here is to treat the pain as early as possible after the patient's presentation. If the pain becomes worse after the administration of pain relief the triage nurse can always up triage the patient.

Haemorrhage

The triage discriminators for haemorrhage are exsanguinating, uncontrolled major and uncontrolled minor. Exsanguinating is obviously a life threat so these patients are allocated a level 1/ red category. The uncontrolled major haemorrhage is defined as bleeding / heavy flow and soaking of the dressings despite large dressings with direct pressure being applied to the wound, these patients are given a level 2 / orange category. The uncontrolled minor haemorrhage is defined as bleeding that is flowing slightly with oozing despite dressings and direct pressure; these patients are given a level 3 / yellow category.

Conscious Level

Adults and children are considered separately in this discriminator, in the adult setting only patients who present fitting are allocated a level 1 / red category. In children all unresponsive children are allocated to this level 1 category. Any adult that has altered consciousness but responds to voice or pain or a child who only responds to voice or pain are allocated a Level 2 / orange which is the very urgent category.

The triage nurse needs to ascertain what has caused the alteration in consciousness so that they can allocate the patient to the correct level of clinical urgency. The nurse must determine if drugs or alcohol are involved, this does not alter their need for treatment or the urgency level allocated. They should be treated no differently to the patient who arrives with an altered conscious state due to a head injury; they both have clinical urgency needs.

Temperature

Temperatures these days can be taken at triage with most triage areas having the tympanic style thermometer. With the MTS system they have developed the skin touch system of a quick form of assessment, very hot skin corresponds to a temperature of > 41°C, hot skin > 38.5°C and warm skin > 37.5°C. An adult that is considered very hot or child with hot skin fits into the very urgent category of level 1/ red, while the adult with hot skin is considered urgent which is level 2 / orange category [9]. Patients that are considered cold temperature < 35°C should also be considered very urgent as they could be septic and very unwell.

Acuteness

This is the term used to assess the patient's illness and some definitions come attached to assist the triage nurse to allocate the patient to the correct level / category.

Abrupt means onset within seconds or minutes, rapid was less than 12 hours, acute describes onset within 12-24 hours and finally recent is sign(s) symptom(s) onset within the past 7 days [9]. This assessment is not designed to place patients that have had symptoms for 7 days or longer to a lower acuity level but the wait these patients have will depend on the workload and acuity in the department.

This is where the ATS system that the author works in is different it does not have these clear discriminators. These discriminators would be a useful tool for any triage nurse to use as a prompting system, allowing them to assess their patients effectively.

The MTS system has a reassessment system called The Manchester Monitor; this is carried out in the waiting room at regular intervals. The need to monitor the patients waiting for treatment does not cease after the initial contact at triage [9]. The triage nurse has the ability to change the triage level / category if the patient's condition deteriorates. In Australia this is called up-triaging the patient. If the triage nurse reassess the patient and decides they need to be seen quicker they can up triage the patient and move them through the department if required. This is what the Manchester Monitor accomplishes as it picks up patient deterioration quickly and acts to rectify the problem if there is one.

The MTS uses patient presentational flow charts with the most common ED presentations that the triage nurse uses, the flow charts come with accompanying notes and the specific discriminators that prompt the triage nurse when questioning the patient allowing them to allocate the patient to the correct triage level. As there are 50 presentational charts it is too difficult to include them in this book, the Emergency Triage book can be purchased from a book store which explains this triage system succinctly. After reading the presentational charts they are very thorough and can be a useful tool for any triage nurse.

CANADIAN TRIAGE AND ACUITY SCALE (CTAS)

The effective management of any (ED) requires a team of highly skilled professional medical and nursing staff [11]. The team must be able to set priorities correctly identifying patient needs, provide appropriate treatment, investigation, and timely disposition [11]. The three important concepts of the CTAS like all triage scales are utility, relevance and validity. The primary objective of the triage scale is timely treatment by a physician, this is because most decisions about investigation and initiation of treatment is made by a physician.

The CTAS is a 5 level triage system used in Canada and abroad which was commenced in 1999 [12]. In 2001 a paediatric version of the CTAS guidelines was developed and published; these guidelines are continually revised by the CTAS National Working Group [12]. The 5 level triage system has times attached to each level and the levels are colour coded.

Level 1 – Resuscitation (colour blue) / continuous care
Level 2 – Emergent (colour red) / 15 minutes
Level 3 – Urgent (colour yellow) / 30 minutes
Level 4 – Less Urgent (colour green) / 60 minutes
Level 5 – Non Urgent (colour white) / 120 minutes

When the patient presents to the triage desk the triage nurse does not only look at the presentation but also looks at the patients condition, pain scale and the signs and symptoms described to assign at triage level. The training required for this triage system must be extensive as the nurse has many factors / modifiers to take into account before assigning a triage level.

The triage nurse must assess the patient's chief complaint looking at why they have presented to the ED and then validate and assess the chief complaint. This is done through a quick 2-5 minute interview / assessment at the triage desk and looks at three areas as follows.

A.   Subjective Data: Onset / Course and Duration

The nurse may have a specific way that they triage patients and not all triage nurses ask questions the same way. The nurse here is asking the patient questions such as

- When did it start?
- How long did it last and does it come and go?
- Is it still present and does it radiate anywhere?
- What relieves the pain or symptoms?
- What is the pain or symptoms like? and finally
- Have you had this before and what was the diagnosis? The triage nurse may also ask the patient their pain scores out of 10 depending what the patient rates their score the nurse will triage them appropriately.

B.   Objective: In this part of the assessment, the nurse decides what area the patient must be treated in.

The triage nurse is looking at the physical appearance of the patient, their skin, general colour (flushed, pink, and cyanotic), the degree of distress the patient is feeling and their emotional responses, anxiousness. Also the nurse may be able to take some vital signs if time allow, these may be necessary when allocating level III, IV and V levels.

C.   Additional Information: Medications

The triage nurse may ask the patient about their current medications they are taking and their past medical history as this may jog the patient memory in regards to medications being taken. An example of this may be the patient stating they take medications for their blood pressure, reflux and nausea [13].

Triage is not a process that is static it is dynamic, meaning that once the patient has been triaged they need to be in an area where the triage nurse can see them and reassess them on a regular basis. The above three points are considered by all triage nurses when they are assessing patients as they present to the triage counter. The CTAS has a system depending on the level given to the patient that states when reassessment should occur. For the level I patient they are continually assessed as they receive continuous care, level II patients should be assessed every 15 minutes, level III every 60 minutes, level IV every 60 minutes and finally level V every 120 minutes [13].

The above intervals are physician assessment times that correspond to the triage levels but nursing reassessment should also occur at these times. Once the nurse has reassessed the patients if they are outside of their allocated triage times for physician assessment "they should be up triaged to avoid unfair bumping and long delays to MD assessment" [13] p7. This differs to the ATS; patients are reassessed and if their condition has changed they will be up triaged to a different category not up triaged as they are outside their allocated time to physician treatment.

The CTAS is a triage system that is quite complicated as the nurse is not only required to allocate a triage level but there are modifiers that must be taken into account, these include pain, respiratory, vital signs, bleeding / haemorrhage to name a few. These are taken into account when the triage nurse is looking at the list of complaint oriented triage (COT). The triage nurse selects from the list and then formulates a triage level after assessing the patient.

So what are the levels of the CTAS? They are discussed below.

Level I – Resuscitation (Blue) / Immediate

This level includes those conditions that are life or limb threatening or imminent risk of deterioration requiring immediate management. Presentations that may be included in the level I presentations are any of the code arrests either cardiac or respiratory including imminent arrest. Major trauma with single or multiple body systems involved, burns involving greater than twenty five percent of the body surface, Glasgow Coma Scale (GCS) less than 10.

Shock states where there is the possibility of imminent arrest, hypotension with either tachycardia or bradycardia [11]. The unconscious patient, this includes patients who are intoxicated or have taken an overdose, all patients who require some form of airway protection or supportive measures and finally patients who have a reversible cause such as those with hypoglycaemia.

Patients with severe respiratory distress who may require support or intervention, including patients with chronic obstructive pulmonary disease (COPD), severe metabolic disturbances such as DKA, chronic heart failure, pulmonary oedema and of course those patients requiring intubation or positive pressure ventilation. As stated before this level one is the same as the other triage systems, anyone presenting with a life threatening illness or at risk of deterioration or death receives care immediately.

Level II – Emergent (Red) / < 15 Minutes

This level deals with patients who have potential threat to life or limb, these are the patients who require rapid medical intervention or the physician can delegate procedures to be commenced. This triage level has many categories of patients that can be allocated, so it can be the one with grey areas where triage nurses may have difficulty deciding whether the patient requires a level 2 or not.

Patients that fit into this level include;

Altered mental states: this can be due to infectious, inflammatory processes, drug effects, poisoning, and metabolic disorders. It can also include those patients with subtle changes such as increased confusion due to no known cause. Young children with irritability and poor feeding can present quite unwell with infections and dehydration. All of these patients should have a blood sugar reading done to exclude hypoglycaemia as the cause as this is easily reversible. If this is the case the triage nurse should reassess the patient once the hypoglycaemia has been treated and re triage the patient.

Head Injury: This is a difficult presentation as it appears in many of the triage levels; patients that present with a GCS less than 13 will require medical review as they may require CT scanning and possibly airway protection. Patients presenting with severe headache, any loss of consciousness, neck symptoms, confusion, or nausea and vomiting will need to be assessed quickly and the appropriate questions asked as to the trauma sustained, time of onset of symptoms and the severity of the symptoms. The triage nurse may ask if the symptoms have changed over a period of time and this is important it gives the triage nurse a chronological timeline of the injury and any deterioration.

Severe Trauma: These patients may present with trauma to a single system or a multiple system involvement but they may have normal vital signs at the time of presentation, if their vital signs are abnormal they are given a level I triage score.

These patients may have moderate to severe pain and will require pain relief quickly.

Neonates: This category of patients come with their own set of complications and this is why they are allocated a level II score, they may show signs of hyperbilirubemia and may have conditions that are not as yet diagnosed. In babies this age there may only be subtle signs of illness but the parents most likely will be very anxious therefore triage nurses should assess these patients very carefully [11]. The triage nurse must listen to the parents concerns as they know their child.

Eye Pain: Any chemical burns (acid or alkali) are given a level II as this is an organ threatening condition, if time to physician treatment could potentially be delayed an assessment by a physician and flushing of the eye can commence. Other conditions that may potentially fit this category may include glaucoma and foreign bodies with increased pain scores.

Chest Pain: This can be one of the most difficult presentations for triage nurses to assess as there can be multiple causes for chest pain. Visceral pain that is lasting can be described as heaviness, squeezing, burning can lead the triage nurse to suspect cardiac chest pain. The triage nurse would also be looking for other cues such as diaphoresis, nausea and vomiting. Sudden sharp chest pain on inspiration may indicate a pulmonary embolism, pneumothorax or even chest wall tenderness. It should also be noted that patients presenting with chest pain that have a prior history of MI, Angina or Pulmonary Embolism (PE) should always be given a level II [11].

Overdose: The patient who takes an intentional overdose is another presentation that the triage nurse may find difficult, trying to obtain a story from an obviously distressed person can be very unreliable. Determining what the patient has taken and exactly how many can be challenging these patients require early physician review as they will require laboratory testing to determine drug levels and if there are any antidotes that may be given. They may also require cardiac monitoring depending on what they have taken. Patients with altered consciousness or vital signs will need to be seen very quickly as they may need to be upgraded to a level I score. Any patient presenting with an overdose in the ATS system are always allocated a priority 2 level.

Abdominal Pain: Patients presenting with abdominal pain will present with varying degrees of pain. Any patient presenting with a pain score of 8/10 or above will require a deeper questioning from the triage nurse as they may have a AAA, an ectopic pregnancy (females 15-50), perforated viscous, appendicitis, bowel obstruction These patients will require prompt physician assessment.

GI Bleed: Patients presenting with GI bleeds (upper or lower) can also be a problem as they have the potential to deteriorate quickly. It must be remembered that one set of normal vital signs does not mean the patient is haemodynamically stable. The triage nurse must ensure these patients are kept within view and have regular vital signs, again, these patients require prompt physician review and commencement of treatment [11]. These patients are given a level II as they have the potential to deteriorate quickly; this is the same with the other triage systems as well.

CVA: As the treatment for CVA improves patients presenting with symptoms suggestive of CVA should be given a level II as they require rapid assessment and commencement of treatment such as CT scan and possibly thrombolysis or surgery if warranted [11]. Patients presenting with these symptoms have a time critical condition they require treatment to commence in less than 4 hours this is the same within the ATS system.

Asthma: The CTAS uses a combination of objective measures to assess asthma, (FEV1, PEFR, and O^2 saturations) although in children under 6years the O^2 saturation is used to estimate the severity. Patients presenting with asthma can be difficult to assess, but if they have had previous serious asthma attacks then the triage nurse should give the patient a level II. Also if the patient can not do the spirometry this should also serves as an indicator that the patient is quite unwell.

Dyspnoea: The problem with patients presenting with dyspnoea it is difficult for the triage nurse to determine if the shortness of breath is due to COPD, asthma, chronic heart failure (CHF), PE, pneumothorax, anaphylaxis or pneumonia or a combination of problems. The triage nurse will need to listen to the patient relaying their story and auscultation of the chest will aid the nurse to make the correct triage decision [11].

Anaphylaxis: This presentation in the ATS is always allocated a priority 2 if there is airway involvement. Using the CTAS it is similar, if there is throat involvement the triage nurse should be suspicious and early adrenaline protocol initiated and a slight delay in physician assessment, particularly if there is a prior history with an uncomplicated course [11]. If able the triage nurse should ascertain what has caused the reaction as true anaphylaxis involves multiple body systems and the compromised patient should be allocated a level II.

Fever: Children less than 3 months with temperatures above 38°C are always allocated a level II. In any age group fever combined with other signs or lethargy, rigors should always have prompt physician assessment as this could be a bacterial infection.

Vomiting and Diarrhoea: If the triage nurse suspect's dehydration especially in paediatric patients they should be allocated a level II. Dehydration in children can be quite serious so close questioning of the parents is vitally important.

Acute psychosis / extreme agitation: The triage nurse must not be judgmental; they need to exclude an organic cause, poisoning or metabolic disturbances. If the psychosis or agitation is part of a known psychiatric illness the patient will require early intervention and possibly medication. Obtaining a history from this patient can be difficult so information from family or other health provider may be all the triage nurse has to go on [11].

Diabetes: These patients may arrive at the triage desk confused with an altered conscious state and the triage nurse must assess them and take a blood sugar level quickly as this will give them vital information. If the patient is hypoglycaemic this can be corrected at triage and then assessed by a physician although if they are high the triage nurse should suspect DKA and the patient allocated a level II and seen by a physician quickly.

Headache: This presentation can appear in a couple of the other triage levels but as a level II the triage nurse is trying to ascertain if the patient has an organ threatening injury or illness such as CVA, TIA, subarachnoid or subdural haemorrhage, meningitis or encephalitis. The patient may have a stress or migraine headache, the triage nurse must question the patient about the onset, duration, intensity, "is this the worst headache you have ever had"? all of these questions will allow the triage nurse to allocate the correct triage level.

Severe Pain: Everybody experiences pain differently and it can be difficult for a triage nurse to assess pain when the patient is stating that it is 8/10 and they look well. The triage nurse in this situation will need to question the patient well in order to make a well informed triage decision. Usually an experienced triage nurse will pick up on the other cues such as facial expression, diaphoresis, body posture which can indicate how much pain the patient is experiencing. The triage nurse must ensure they are not judgemental and offer the patient pain relief as soon as possible.

Abuse/neglect/assault: This group of patients may not have life threatening injuries but in the case of sexual assault there is the time critical factor of 4 hours, these patients should be given a level II as they will require assessment and the collection of evidence. Other assault patients can be given a level III depending on their injuries; this is at the discretion of the triage nurse and their assessment.

Immunocompromised: These patients may present febrile post chemotherapy, or they may have a condition that immunocompromises them such as HIV, a malignancy, a known immune deficiency, or on medication. These patients are at a higher risk than others so should be isolated and will require early assessment.

These are just some of the level II presentations and as mentioned before some of these presentations can be seen in the other levels. It is difficult to demonstrate what fits into a level II category and that is why the CTAS has the COT list for the triage nurse to use if required. I have specifically explained all of these presentations and why the CTAS has them as a level 2, the reason being is that in any of the other triage systems the nurses are also using these types of discriminators and in many of the triage systems they are allocated the same triage level.

Level III Urgent (Yellow) / < 30 Minutes

Patients that fit into this CTAS level are those who require urgent treatment as their condition may progress requiring more urgent intervention. Patients in this level may be in considerable pain and not be able to attend work or function as they normally would.

Patients that fit into this level include;

Head Injury: These patients should have a GCS of 15 and a pain score of less than 8/10 to qualify for a CTAS level III, if the triage nurse feels the patient does not meet this standard they can allocate a level II score and have the patient seen in a timelier manner.

Moderate trauma: These are the patients that present with fractures or simple sprains and dislocations that can be administered pain relief and wait a little longer to see a physician. Dislocations should be reduced promptly in less than 30 minutes so physician assessment should occur within this time [11].

Asthma: As mentioned in the level II category some asthma patients are able to wait a little longer to see a physician, if their FEV1 or PEFR is greater than 60 percent and their O^2 saturations are greater that 95 percent these patients can wait for 30 minutes to see a physician. They must be placed into an area where the triage nurse can see them and reassessment can occur, if the triage nurse feels the patient requires up triaging they can facilitate this [11].

Shortness of Breath: Patients that are allocated a level III with shortness of breath are those with pneumonia, URTI's and COPD. The triage nurse should have assessed the O^2 saturations and if concerned up triage the patients or they should be in an area where they can be viewed and reassessed frequently.

Chest Pain: In the level III classification these are the patients who present with sharp pain may be pain on inspiration or coughing. This is not considered cardiac type chest pain, if the triage nurse suspects cardiac chest pain especially in the elderly that can be poor historians they should be a level II triage score. The rest of these types of patients are considered to be experiencing chest wall pain or pain that is pulmonary and pleuritic in nature.

Vaginal bleeding / GI bleeding: With both of these types of bleeding the patient can be unstable so they require regular vital signs and be placed into an area where they can be viewed by the triage nurse at all times. If their vital signs are stable they can wait 30 minutes for physician assessment although the triage nurse can up triage the patients at any time if their condition deteriorates.

Acute Pain: Pain is the most frequent reason for patients presenting to the ED, patients in the level III category frequently present with renal colic, migraine headache, and back pain. The triage nurse must assess the pain score and make the decision as to whether the patient can wait for physician assessment or requires up triage. A pain score of approximately 4-7/10 is appropriate for this level; triage nurse can obtain orders for pain relief prior to physician assessment.

Level IV Semi-Urgent (Green) < 60 Minutes

Patients allocated a triage level IV are those that are either distressed, and have the potential for deterioration or those who benefit from intervention or reassurance within 60-120 minutes [11].

Head Injury: If a patient presents with a GCS of 15, and the trauma occurred 4-6 hours ago and they symptoms have not changed since the time of the accident, they can wait 60 minutes for physician assessment.

Minor Trauma: Sprains, minor fractures, laceration, abrasions, contusions who have a pain score of 4-7/10 meet this triage level.

Abdominal pain: Acute intensity pain of 4-7/10, or a child that is not too distressed. Patient has normal vital signs and the patient does not look distressed. These are the patients with constipation, early appendicitis.

Headache: These are the patients who present with no high risk associated symptoms; they may have sinusitis, URTI, or flu like illness. Vital signs should be normal.

Ear ache. Otitis media or externa can give the patient sufficient pain that they would present to the ED a pain score of 4-7/10, the triage nurse can obtain an order for pain relief to be administered prior to physician assessment.

Corneal foreign body: Patient with no change to their visual acuity and a mild or moderate pain score fit this triage level.

Back pain, chronic: These patients must be treated as though this is a new onset of back pain, meaning the triage nurse must question the patient closely so that symptoms are not missed and the patient does not suffer any serious outcomes. If the symptoms are the same as their usual back pain they can wait to see a physician.

Upper Respiratory Tract Infections: This is another frequent presentation to the ED, a patient arrives stating they have a sore throat, cough, fever; nasal congestion can wait to see a physician. The triage nurse must assess the patient thoroughly to exclude anything more serious such as strep throat, peritonsillar abscess [11].

These are just some of the presentations that can be allocated a triage level IV in the CTAS triage system. These presentations are similar to the category 4 presentations in the ATS system.

Level V Non Urgent (White) < 120 Minutes

Like most of the other triage systems examined, patients allocated a level V triage score are those that may be part of a chronic problem that shows either no or some deterioration. These patients could be referred to general practitioners (or other parts of the health system).

Minor trauma: tendonitis, abrasions, wound care, immunisations, nursing interventions.

Sore throat, URTI: Minor viral illnesses, low grade fever in adults.

Vaginal bleeding: Normal menses or postmenopausal bleeding in patients with normal vital signs and low pain score.

Psychiatric: These are the patients who are having difficulty obtaining care from other health care providers, they may have minor problems [11], the triage nurse must be sensitive to these patients' problems as they may have no where else to go. This is the patient who has chronic depression or chronic psychiatric disturbances.

The CTAS system of triaging is complicated as it uses flow charts, (similar to the MTS system), the nurse assesses the patient but they also use the complaint orientated triage (COT) flow charts to guide them. The above information has been taken from the Implementation Guidelines for CTAS. Information about the Complaint Oriented Triage (COTS) and other information about the CTAS can be accessed from www.caep.ca. Nurses using the CTAS system of triage would be required to undergo a training course that covers not only triaging and how it works but also how to use the COTS system. Being a triage nurse requires expertise and a sound knowledge base so using the CTAS would in my opinion require the nurse to have many years of ED nursing behind them.

All of the above triage systems have their own individual ways of allocating the triage score, the ESI uses acuity level and resources, the CTAS and MTS use presentational charts and complaint orientated triage charts. The ATS does not have these types of charts to work from; also the education of triage nurses around the world is different. The MTS, ESI and CTAS all have lengthy training programs attached to them. The ATS does vary from hospital to hospital depending on their policies have a shorter training system. In the hospital the author works in the triage orientation is quite short and requires the completion of a training package and two days orientation to triage.

ATTRIBUTES OF A TRIAGE NURSE

The triage nurse is the first person the patient encounters when they present to the emergency department and there are some attributes that all triage nurses should possess in order to perform the role well. The triage nurse must have a diverse knowledge base as they will be presented with many situations and must be able to problem solve using past experiences and their knowledge of emergency nursing. They must also have the ability to make a rapid decision based on the information provided by the patient; this decision must be accurate and not place the patient at risk.

The triage nurse must possess excellent communication skills and strong interpersonal skills, triage nurses must be strong communicators as triage is an area where communication is vital. Communication is both verbal and nonverbal at triage and the triage nurse must be aware of how they present themselves to the public and what nonverbal cues they may be sending the patient as they register. The triage nurse must have excellent physical assessment skills as these are used at triage to assess patients as they present. This is one of the most important skills of the triage nurse, the triage nurse may decide to listen to a patient's chest and they must understand what they are hearing and what it means for the patient as this will affect the triage priority assigned.

Critical thinking skills are a requirement of the triage nurse and the importance of critical thinking is explained in the next chapter. Hand in hand with critical thinking comes the ability to conduct a focussed and brief interview at triage, the triage nurse has approximately 3 minutes to ascertain why the patient has presented to the ED. Information provided in this interview by the patient is used to assign a clinical triage priority. The triage nurse must be able to select the appropriate information provided by the patient, analyse the information and assign the correct triage priority. These critical thinking skills at triage are vital and play an important role in assigning the correct triage priority for that particular patient presentation.

The triage nurse must also possess the ability to work under periods of stress, and during stressful situations. This is a very important attribute as the triage nurse may have to work during conditions where there is an increased number patient presentations and overcrowding in the ED. When working in an area where there is an increased period of stress the triage nurse must be able to multitask and delegate and these are another two important attributes to have. The triage nurse cannot perform every role and must be able to delegate to other staff tasks that are required in the triage area such as administering pain relief, slings, and simple dressings.

The triage nurse must have a good understanding in regards to cultural and religious diversity as they may have patients presenting to the ED from diverse cultural backgrounds. The triage nurse does not want to offend anyone when they are trying to register and they are unwell, so variations in practice may have to occur. An example of this may be a gentleman presenting with urinary retention and due to cultural differences cannot discuss this issue with a female triage nurse, the triage nurse may have to find a male doctor or male triage competent nurse to triage this patient. Triaging the patient is about obtaining the correct information which allows the triage nurse to assign the correct triage priority, if the patient is reluctant to provide information the triage nurse should show compassion and try and make the patient comfortable so they can receive the correct treatment.

The triage nurse must have sound patient education skills; sometimes the triage counter provides an excellent opportunity for the triage nurse to provide education to the patient. The patient may have presented to the ED with chest pain when they should have called an ambulance, the triage nurse could advise the patient about the importance of calling an ambulance as the crew can commence treatment immediately.

There are a few more attributes of the triage nurse that must be mentioned and these include being compassionate, caring, understanding, and sound knowledge about customer service

REFERENCES

[1]   Oxford Online Dictionary, http://oxforddictionaries.com/, downloaded on 24th January 2013.

[2]   Ganley. L, Gloster.AS (2011) An overview of triage in the (ED) *Nursing Standard* , vol 26, No 12, pp 49-56

[3]   Lahdet. Eric Fortes (2009) Analysis of Triage worldwide. *Emergency Nurse* Vol 17, No 4, pp 16-19

[4]   Farronhknia. Nasin, et al (2011) (ED) Triage Scales and their Components: A Systematic review of the Scientific Evidence. *Scandinavian Journal of Trauma, resuscitation and Emergency Medicine* Vol 19, No 42, pp 1-13

[5]   Towomcy. M, Lcc.A ct at (2012) Limitations in validating (ED) triage scales. *Emergency Medicine Journal* Vol 24, pp 477-479

[6]   Janssen. Maaike, Van Achterberg, Theo et al (2011) Adherence to the guideline "triage in (ED)s": a survey of Dutch (ED)s. *Journal of Clinical Nursing Vol 20, pp 2458-2468*

[7]   Australian Government, Department of Health and Ageing (2007) Emergency Triage Education Kit. Canberra. ACT

[8]   Yousif. Khalid, Bebbington, Jane et al (2005) Impact on patients triage distribution using the Australasian triage Scale compared with its predecessor the National Triage Scale. *Emergency Medicine Australasia* Vol 17, pp 429-433

[9]   Manchester Triage Group. *Emergency Triage*, 2nd Edition, Blackwell Publishing, BMJ Books. (2006)

[10]   Agency for Healthcare Research and Quality, Emergency Severity Index (ESI) A Triage Tool for (ED) Care. Version 4. Implementation handbook. 2012 Edition

[11]   1998. Implementation Guidelines for the Canadian (ED) Triage & Acuity Scale *(CTAS)*. Downloaded 19/1/2013 from http://caep.ca/resources/ctas

[12]   Bullard M.J, Unger B, et al. 2008. Revisions to the Canadian (ED) Triage and Acuity Scale (CTAS) adult guidelines. *Canadian Journal of Emergency*

Medicine, March 2008; 10 (2), pp 136-42. Downloaded 19/1/2013 from http://caep.ca/resources/ctas

[13] Meek. Robert, Wilson. Phiri (2005) Australasian Triage Scale: Consumer perspective *Emergency Medicine Australasia,* (17) pp 212-217

Chapter 3

CRITICAL THINKING

ABSTRACT

This chapter deals with critical thinking and higher order thinking required to make decisions in regards to patient care. Triage nurses are the first person the patient meets when they present to the (ED). The nurse asks the patient questions which gives them a snapshot of why the patient has presented. From this snapshot the nurse makes a decision as to what priority the patient receives. This priority decides how quickly the patient must be seen by a doctor. How does the nurse make these decisions? What processes does she/he go through in making these decisions?

INTRODUCTION

The ability to think outside the square is very important when making decisions about patient care at triage. The triage nurse is the first person the patient encounters on presentation to the (ED). The triage nurse greets the patient and usually the first question asked is "What has bought you to the (ED) today?" It is the triage nurse who makes the decision on what priority the patient receives. This means the nurse listens to the patient story and then makes an informed decision as to how quickly the patient should be seen.

It is this decision that can influence the outcome of the patient's journey. The decision made by the triage nurse will depend on many factors such as the patient's story, clinical / visual presentation and clinical vital signs. The triage nurse collates all of these findings and makes a decision as to the priority of urgency that the patient should receive. This correlates to how quickly the patient needs to be seen by a doctor.

The triage nurse is a highly skilled and experienced registered nurse who has the ability to collate the information given by the patient into a triage priority or category. It is this higher order thinking or critical thinking that is important to giving the patient the appropriate triage priority.

CRITICAL THINKING – SO WHAT IS IT?

Edwards 2007 has described critical thinking as being very relevant to nursing practice, it is used when situations arise where there is no definitive answer, for example at triage where there is no right or wrong triage score. The nurse weighs up all the information provided by the patient, collates the information quickly, thinks about all the possible variables and makes a decision as to the appropriate triage score required for that patient. The triage nurse relies on past nursing experience and critical thinking to analyse the information provided by the patient and then assign the appropriate triage priority.

Critical thinking has been related to the nursing process. In literature critical thinking can be labelled by many different terms, *i.e.* clinical reasoning, clinical judgement, problem solving and decision making. All of these terms can be used interchangeably [2] It is important for a nurse to have sound clinical reasoning or critical thinking skills as nurses with these skills make positive impacts on patient care [2]. Therefore it can be assumed those with poorly developed clinical reasoning skills have a potentially negative impact on patient outcomes.

So what is critical thinking, and why do nurses need to have these skills so badly in order to perform their roles and provide safe, effective care for their patients. There has been a lot of work done around what critical thinking actually is. Nurses use critical thinking skills every day, skills such as reflecting, clarifying, analysing and reasoning [3]. Nurses use the nursing process to assess, analyse / diagnose, plan, implement and evaluate the care provided to their patients.

There have been many definitions as to what critical thinking is, Chaffe 2003 defined critical thinking as "making sense of our world by carefully examining the thinking process in order to clarify and improve our understanding" [3]. Faccione 1990 has suggested that critical thinking needs the nurse to have the ability to discriminate relevant from the irrelevant information [4]. Brix [5] states "critical thinking is an essential and ongoing process in using theory to guide nursing practice". At triage the nurse uses these critical thinking skills as Brix has said to discriminate the relevant form the irrelevant information provided by the patient in order to assign the correct triage priority.

I always say to new triage nurses listen carefully to what the patient is saying and pick out the important parts of the story, as triage nurses we do not need to know what they had for breakfast or dinner the previous three days but we do need to know the patient has vomited after every meal and has a constant burning in his stomach. Here the triage nurse must pick out the relevant parts of the patient story, and that is he vomits after every meal and may have a stomach or peptic ulcer, it is this ability to think critically that is required at triage.

New graduates are very good at critical thinking as they have been taught and used the process during their studies. New graduates use this beginning level of critical thinking whereas nurses on the floor with more experience used a more advanced level of critical thinking in their everyday practice [5]. This is due to their experiential / situational learning and their expanded knowledge in regards to nursing literature.

So let's look at the nursing process, this is a process that both beginning and experienced nurses use to examine important information about the patient they are caring for [6]. What are the steps in the nursing process?

- The nurse gathers the data about the patient,
- The nurse examines the data and formulates an nursing diagnosis,
- The nurse then formulates a plan of care,
- Care plan is implemented,
- The care is evaluated and finally
- The care is revised and any changes to the care are made [6].

Every nurse uses the nursing process in the care they provide their patients each day. They initially assess their patients, they gather the data, and from this data they formulate a nursing diagnosis. Care is then planned for this patient, the nurse implements and then evaluates the care provided, the nurse then either continues with the same care plan or they revise and make changes to the care.

This is not dissimilar to what occurs at triage when a patient presents to the triage desk. The triage nurse will assess the patient and from that story they formulate a nursing diagnosis and assign a triage priority. It is this nursing diagnosis that decides the treatment path or plan of care. From here the patient may be cared for by nurses in the main department so the process starts again. The nursing process is a dynamic, evolving process that is always being evaluated, and plans of care changed.

Critical thinking plays as important role in conjunction with the nursing process. The nursing process encourages nurses to think systematically which assists them to process the information provided by the patient [6]. It is this systematic thinking process that enables the nurse to obtain objective, subjective, historical and clinical data. The nursing process has some common themes with critical thinking but they are not exactly the same thing. Problem solving requires critical thinking and analysis, the nurse uses these skills to provide the patient with an effective plan of care.

Nurses at triage need to be critical thinkers, they need to be able to quickly analyse what they are seeing in front of them and make a decision as to how quickly the patient requires care to be commenced. The triage nurse is responsible for assessing and screening the patients prior to them being allocated a bed in a treatment area. The triage nurse has to make decisions with limited information and relies on what visual cues they are seeing when the patient is relaying their story and this can be very difficult [7].

Triage nurses are generally nurses who have worked in the ED for quite a few years prior to their triage training, so they have a sound knowledge base and good clinical skills. Many triage nurses have worked in the emergency field of nursing 5-10 years or more. These nurses have undertaken specialised training and triage education in order to equip them with the skills to perform the triage role.

When a patient presents to the triage window with chest pain for example the triage nurse will greet them and ask why they have presented to the ED. The nurse has asked their first question but they have gained quite a lot of visual information. They have seen the patient walk to the desk, they have heard the patient answer their first question. A great deal of information can be obtained from this initial encounter, the nurse can see if the patient is short of breath, diaphoretic, grimacing or holding their chest.

The triage nurse will then ask as many questions as they feel is required to enable them to make an informed decision. From the verbal answers given by the patient and from all of the visual and clinical information the triage nurse will be analysing and formulating a nursing diagnosis. The triage nurse after formulating a nursing diagnosis will rule out all of the possible differential diagnoses that could be the cause of the chest. It is this critical thinking that the triage nurse uses to decide on a triage priority / level assigned to the patient.

The triage interview which lasts approximately 3-5 minutes is all the time the triage nurse has to obtain as much information as possible in order for them to formulate a nursing diagnosis which leads to a triage level or category. The triage nurse must use the information to assign the triage category ensuring the category assigned is correct. At triage there is a chance that the nurse might either under or over triage the patient and this is not what triage is all about. Triage is about assigning a priority commensurate with the acuity of the patients presenting complaint.

The experience of the triage nurse plays an important role here although all nurses are prone to over and under triaging patients. This is the reason triage education plays a vital role; nurses must have had comprehensive education in order to perform the role of triage effectively. With this education and their experience the triage nurse will use their critical thinking skills to allocate the patient to the correct triage priority. Education provided to triage nurses will depend on the individual hospital's policies and procedures.

Triage nurses are expected to make sound clinical decisions in a time pressured environment and require the knowledge base in regards to signs and symptoms of disease. This is why it is important that nurses who are chosen to undertake triage education have many years of nursing and ED nursing experience. They use critical thinking to justify decisions made based on the clinical, physiological and patient history provided at the triage desk by the patient.

The triage nurse must be able to sift through information provided by the patient then prioritise the information formulating a triage priority / level. Critical thinking and clinical expertise plays a vital part in the triage nurse being able to perform their role effectively. Every nurse on every shift they work use critical thinking to care for their patient clinical decision making is an important part of every day nursing practice. Making the correct clinical decisions can sometimes have life altering effects so the correct decision made at the right time is important.

REFERENCES

[1] Edwards. S (2007) Critical thinking: A two-phase framework. *Nursing Education Practice.* 2007 (7), pp 303-314

[2] University of Newcastle (2009) Clinical reasoning Instructor Resources. School of Nursing and Midwifery, faculty of Health. *University of Newcastle*

[3] Nugent. P M, Vitale. B A (2008) in Test success: Test taking techniques for beginning Nursing Students. 5th edn F A Davis Company 2008

[4] Edwards. S (2003) critical thinking at the bedside: a practical perspective. *British Journal of Nursing* Vol 12, No 19 ,pp 1142-49

[5] Clarke Brix. E (1993) critical thinking and theory based practice *Holistic Nursing Practice* Vol 7, No 3, pp 21-27

[6] Huckabay, Loucine (2009) Clinical Reasoned Judgement and the Nursing Process. *Nursing Forum* Vol 44, No 2, April – June 2009, pp 72-78

[7] Australian Government, Department of Health and Ageing (2007) Emergency Triage Education Kit. Canberra. ACT

Chapter 4

CASE STUDIES AND ANSWERS

ABSTRACT

Chapter four has case studies with the expected answers supplied at the back of the chapter. These case studies are of presentations that the nurse may deal with in a triage context and prompt the nurse to problem solve their way through the case presentation and allocate a triage score / priority. These case studies have been chosen to prompt the beginning triage nurse to use their training and clinical skills to decide on what category to allocate the patient.

INTRODUCTION

This chapter deals with some case studies that the nurse can work through and allocate a triage priority / level to the patient. The expected answers and rationale are at the back of the chapter. The author has used the information provided by the triage systems and has allocated a triage score that they feel meets the patient presentation. It must be remembered that there is no right or wrong answer when allocating a triage score.

The four triage systems used are the ATS, CTAS, ESI and the MTS, they all require training and expertise to use them effectively, the author has used the ATS and has used information available at the websites in the previous chapter the allocate triage categories to the patient scenarios.

CASE STUDIES

1. A 40 year old male presents to the triage counter and states; he is having a heavy sensation in his chest that is radiating to his right shoulder. He looks in pain, has small beads of sweat on his forehead and appears slightly short of breath. You take his pulse and it is 115 beats per minute. This man is also noted to be slightly overweight.

   a) What questions do you ask this patient?
   b) What is your nursing diagnosis?
   c) What priority / triage score do you give this patient? Circle your answer below.

1	2	3	4	5

Now check your answers at the back of the chapter.

2. A mother brings her 1 year old child to the triage window and states; the baby has been unwell for 3 days with a high temperature, runny nose and she is unsettled and crying all the time. She won't eat and is not drinking a lot. The child looks flushed with reddened cheeks and feels warm to touch. You notice she is breathing rapidly and has a tracheal tug and mild rib recession. You take her respiratory rate and it is 44 breaths per minute, her temperature is 38.3° C / 100.94 Fahrenheit.

   a) What questions would you ask this mother?
   b) What is your nursing diagnosis?
   c) What priority / triage score would you give this baby? Circle your answer below

1	2	3	4	5

Now check your answers at the back of the chapter.

3. A young man presents to the triage counter limping on his right leg. He states he has hurt his ankle playing soccer. You notice he is quite swollen on the lateral side of the right ankle.

    a) What questions do you ask the young man?
    b) What is your nursing diagnosis?
    c) What priority / triage score to you give him? Circle your answer below

1	2	3	4	5

Now check your answers at the back of the chapter.

4. An elderly gentleman presents to the triage window with his wife saying that she has been vomiting for 3 days and has diarrhoea for the past 2 days. He is worried as she has a heart condition and can not keep her medication down. Her pulse is 130 beats per minute and irregular, she is actively vomiting and states she feels terrible.

    a) What questions do you ask this couple?
    b) What is your nursing diagnosis?
    c) What priority / triage score do you give this lady? Circle your answer below.

1	2	3	4	5

Now check your answers at the back of the chapter.

5. A 45 year old man presents to triage stating that he has splashed a chemical in his right eye. He has washed the eye out for 10 minutes with cool running tap water but he can still feel it burning.

    a) What questions do you ask this man?
    b) What is your nursing diagnosis?
    c) What priority / triage score do you give this man? Circle your answer below.

1	2	3	4	5

Now check your answers at the back of the chapter.

6. A young man presents to the ED complaining of shortness of breath and chest pain in his right upper chest. The young man is tall and lanky, and he states the pain came on suddenly and is sharp in nature.

    a) What questions do you ask this man?
    b) What is your nursing diagnosis?
    c) What priority / triage score do you give her? Circle your answer below

1	2	3	4	5

Now check your answers at the back of the chapter.

7. A young woman presents to triage stating she is 8 weeks pregnant; she has lower abdominal pain and some spotting.

    a) What questions do you ask this lady?
    b) What is your nursing diagnosis?
    c) What priority / triage score do you give her? Circle your answer below

1	2	3	4	5

Now check your answers at the back of the chapter.

8. A lady presents to triage with her 2 year old daughter saying she will not use her left arm. Her arm is hanging beside her body limply.

    a) What questions do you ask this mother?
    b) What is your nursing diagnosis?
    c) What priority / triage score do you give her? Circle your answer below

1	2	3	4	5

Now check your answers at the back of the chapter.

9. A young lady presents after playing basketball stating she has hurt her left knee. The knee looks visibly swollen and she is walking with a moderate limp.

    a) What questions do you ask this lady?
    b) What is your nursing diagnosis?
    c) What priority / triage score do you give her? Circle your answer below

1	2	3	4	5

Now check your answers at the back of the chapter.

10. A man presents to triage stating he has a painful hand. The hand is very swollen and bruised looking and there are some grazes over the 4th and 5th knuckles.

    a) What questions do you ask this lady?
    b) What is your nursing diagnosis?
    c) What priority / triage score do you give her? Circle your answer below

1	2	3	4	5

Now check your answers at the back of the chapter.

11. A young lady presents stating she has missed her appointment with her local doctor and needs a prescription for the oral contraceptive pill.

    a) What questions do you ask this lady?
    b) What is your nursing diagnosis?
    c) What priority / triage score do you give her? Circle your answer below

1	2	3	4	5

Now check your answers at the back of the chapter.

12. A young woman presents to the triage counter stating she is 28 weeks pregnant and she is having abdominal pain, it is her first baby and she is worried something is wrong with the baby.

   a)   What questions do you ask this lady?
   b)   What is your nursing diagnosis?
   c)   What priority / triage score do you give her? Circle your answer below

1	2	3	4	5

Now check your answers at the back of the chapter.

13. A 60 year old man presents to the triage desk stating he fell over last night hitting the left side of his chest on a chair. He is pale and sweaty looking, he states he can not take a deep breath in as he experiences a sharp pain in his left chest. His respiratory rate is shallow and a little quick. You notice he is holding the left side of his chest.

   a)   What questions do you ask this man?
   b)   What is your nursing diagnosis?
   c)   What priority / triage score do you give him? Circle your answer below

1	2	3	4	5

Now check your answers at the back of the chapter.

ANSWERS

Case Study One

a) What questions do you ask?

   I.   Do you have any pre-existing medical conditions?

      You ask this question to try and elicit information from the patient about his past medical history. The patient has presented to the (ED) with chest pain so you need to know does he have hypertension, a pre-existing heart condition such as angina, previous myocardial infarction (MI), hypercholesterolemia or a rhythm disturbance. You are also trying to find out if the patient has had any major surgeries in the past that could be causing the chest pain. All of these answers will affect the triage decision that you make.

II. Do you have any family history of heart disease?

The reason that you ask this question is to try and find out if this patient is at risk of heart disease due to the familial connections. Here you are trying to find out if the patient has either parents or siblings with heart disease. You also ask are they still alive and well or at what age did they die. Most patients will elicit this information freely.

III. Where is the pain? Do you have the pain now?

The reason this question is asked is you are trying to determine is the pain cardiac / respiratory / musculoskeletal. The patient has told you he has central chest pain radiating to the right shoulder. So we need to know does it radiate anywhere else, such as the left arm, the right arm or the jaw. It must be noted that one patient's chest pain when experiencing an MI or angina is not the same as the next patient, there is no real classical signs for MI. You ask the patient if they have the pain now and what relieves it if anything. They may have had the pain an hour ago but now it is just heaviness, this does not exclude MI or angina.

IV. Does it hurt when you take a deep breath in?

The reason for asking this question is to try and determine if the cause for the chest pain is respiratory in nature; such as pneumothorax, pleurisy or chest infection / pneumonia.

V. How long have you had the pain?

This is an important question as you may have heard the saying "time is heart muscle" If the pain is cardiac in nature then your nursing diagnosis and triage priority / score is important.

VI Are you on any regular medications?

This is an important question as it may allude to the cause of the chest pain.

If the patient tells you he is on aspirin, nitrates, statins and antihypertensives this will no doubt make you think cardiac chest pain. If he tells you he is on antibiotics, pain relieving medications you may be thinking respiratory in nature. A word of caution here if you gut is still telling you this patient needs to be seen quickly then either ask a doctor or give them a triage priority / score that reflects the patients urgency.

b) What is your nursing diagnosis?
Chest pain that is cardiac in nature can not be ruled out.

c) What triage category do you give this patient?
ATS – 2 (patient must be seen within 10 minutes)
CTAS – 2 (3 emergent within 15 minutes)
MTS – 2 (very urgent within 10 minutes)
ESI – 2 (Should begin immediately)

Case Study Two

a) What questions do you ask?
I. How long has the child been unwell?
    The reason you are asking this question is you are trying to ascertain if the child has just become unwell today or has been unwell for many days as this can affect the triage score you assign this child. If the child has been unwell for many days he/she may be dehydrated, and beginning to decompensate and require care quickly.
II. How many days has the child had a high temperature?
    This is also an important question as it provides information as to how long the child has had the illness. Also this question should be followed by has any medication such as paracetamol or ibuprofen been administered and has it had an effect on reducing the temperature.
III. When was the last time the baby ate and drank properly? When was the baby's last wet nappy?
    This will along with assessing the baby give the triage nurse an idea of whether the baby is dehydrated. So the question about the wet nappies is also important as this will give you information about the child's hydration status. If the baby has not had a wet nappy for 24 hours at the age of 12 months the child could be quite dehydrated.
IV. Is there any history of breathing problems?
    This question is asked as children of this age group can suffer from noisy breathing, bronchiolitis, respiratory syncytial virus (respiratory virus causing bronchiolitis and respiratory tract infections).
V. Any past medical history?
    This is an important question as it may give the triage nurse an idea as to whether this is a recurring illness. The nurse may ask if the baby was

born at term as this can give you an idea to any pre-existing medical conditions. It is also important to know if the child has any pre-existing cardiac conditions.

VI. Has the child seen a medical professional in the last couple of days?
This is an important question as the child may have seen their local doctor who may have commenced antibiotics or some other medication. This will give the triage nurse an idea as to whether medication and treatment has been commenced and is it effective.

b) What is your nursing diagnosis?

It could be a number of conditions such as Bronchiolitis, Upper / Lower Respiratory Tract Infection or even Pneumonia.

c) What triage category / score do you give this patient?
ATS – 3 (30 minutes)
CTAS – Level 3 (30 minutes)
MTS – Level 3 (60 minutes)
ESI – Level-2

Case Study Three

a) What questions do you ask this patient?
I. What was the mechanism of the injury?
This is an important question as it will give some information as to the type of injury that may have occurred. Was it an inversion or eversion injury? The reason for asking this question as the injury may also involve the foot.
II. Did the ankle swell up immediately?
This will give you an idea as to whether it may be a fracture or ligamentous in nature of course you will not know for sure until the patient has had radiographs done.
III. Have you injured this ankle before?
The patient may have had ligamentous injuries to this ankle before so he may have weak ankles. Also it is important to know if the patient has fractured this ankle before, and if they have any pins and plates in the ankle.

IV. Have you taken any pain relief?

This is important as before the doctor or nurse practitioner examines the patient he may require some pain relief. So it is important to know if he has already self medicated with analgesia.

b) What is your nursing diagnosis?

Sprain / Strain to ankle ligaments.

? Fracture of the ankle or the base on the 5th metatarsal of the foot.

c) What is your triage priority / score?

ATS – 5 (120 minutes)

CTAS – 5 (120 minutes)

MTS – 4 (120 minutes)

ESI – Level-4 (requires one resource)

Case Study Four

a) What questions do you ask?

I. How long have you been unwell?

The reason for asking this question is this patient is elderly with a cardiac condition and she has been experiencing gastroenteritis like symptoms for 3-4 days. The triage nurse is trying to elicit information as to how dehydrated the patient is and whether she is managing to keep her cardiac medications down. This question will also give the triage nurse some information as to how sick the patient is likely to be.

II. What cardiac condition do you have?

This is an important question as the triage nurse needs to know if the patient has cardiac condition that involves a rhythm disturbance, angina or previous MI.

III. What medications are you currently taking?

This question is very important as the patient may be taking anti-arrhythmic medication which if she has gastroenteritis will not be absorbed. Also the medication profile will give the triage nurse information as to how serious the patient's cardiac condition actually is.

IV. Are you keeping anything down?

This question is important as the triage nurse can ascertain how dehydrated the patient is and if there is any chances the patient may have electrolyte disturbances. This is very important as patients with cardiac conditions who have electrolyte imbalances are a greater risk of adverse outcomes.

V. Have you seen your general practitioner about this illness?

The reason for asking this question is the patient may have sought medical advice early on in the illness and their condition has worsened. It is also important as the general practitioner may have commenced them on some medications and it is important to know what the patient has already tried to ameliorate their symptoms.

b) What is your nursing diagnosis?

Gastroenteritis

Viral gastroenteritis

Food poisoning

c) What triage category / score do you give this patient?

ATS – 2 (10 minutes)

CTAS – 3 (30 minutes)

MTS – 3 (60 minutes)

ESI – Level-3 (requires two or more resources)

Case Study Five

a) What questions do you ask?

I. Do you know what the name of the chemical that has splashed your eye?

The reason for asking this question is you need to know if the chemical is an acid or an alkaloid solution. This will assist the doctor in the management of the burn.

II. How long have you rinsed your eye for?

It is important to know if the eye has received a good rinse out with cool water to dilute the chemical.

III. Have you ever injured this eye before?

This important to know as when the doctor examines the eye he can determine what is new / old damage to the cornea.

IV. What is the pain in your eye like on a scale of 0 (being no pain) and 10 (being the worst pain ever) what would you score your pain level?

This question is important as the patient will undoubtedly require pain relief and the level of pain will dictate what pain relief you administer the patient. The other question here is; have they already taken pain relief prior to presentation to the ED.

b) What is your nursing diagnosis?

Chemical burn to the left eye.

c) What triage category / score do you give this patient?

ATS – 2 (10 minutes)

CTAS – 2 (15 minutes)

MTS – 1 (immediate)

ESI - Level -2 (limb or organ threatening condition)

Case Study Six

a) What questions do you ask this patient?

I. Where exactly is the pain, does it radiate anywhere, is it constant and what type of pain is it?

It is important to find out exactly where the pain is and if it radiates anywhere else in the chest, as it could be cardiac in nature. Also here you are looking to see if the pain comes and goes or is there constantly. How the patient describes their pain is also important as it may lead you to suspect different origins for the pain.

II. Is the pain worse on inspiration or expiration?

This question is important as the nurse is narrowing the causes for the pain. Pain on inspiration / expiration will lead the nurse to suspect respiratory causes for the chest pain.

III. Did the pain come on suddenly or over a period of time?

Patients who have a spontaneous pneumothorax will experience sudden pain and by asking this question the nurse is narrowing their suspicions for the cause of the pain.

b) What is your nursing diagnosis?

Pneumothorax

Upper Respiratory Tract Infection

c) What triage category / score do you give this patient?
    ATS – 2 (10 minutes)
    CTAS – 3 (30 minutes)
    MTS – 3 (60 minutes)
    ESI – Level -2

Case Study Seven

a) What questions do you ask this lady?
   I.   How long have you had the pain?
         The patient has explained that she has lower abdominal pain, it is
         important to know if the pain has just started or has she had the pain for a
         couple of days. This will give the triage nurse information as to whether
         the patient could be having a miscarriage.
   II.   How much spotting have you had?
         This question is asked along with how frequently you are changing the
         sanitary pads. This information will give the triage nurse information
         about how much bleeding the patient is experiencing and will also give
         the nurse an idea of their haemodynamic status. The patient could already
         be miscarrying and require additional support such as IV fluids.
   III. Do you have any shoulder tip pain or upper abdominal pain?
         This question is very important as it may allude to the possibility of
         ectopic pregnancy. A patient with this type of pain can deteriorate quite
         quickly and will require treatment in a timely manner.
   IV.   Has the pregnancy been confirmed by your local doctor?
         This is important as the patient may not actually be pregnant? It is
         important to ask this question as it gives the nurse information about care
         provided prior to presentation. The patient may have had the pregnancy
         confirmed on blood test or ultrasound and this information is important. It
         is still important to test the urine for beta HCG to confirm pregnancy in
         the ED. If the pregnancy has been confirmed on ultrasound then this will
         rule out ectopic pregnancy.
   V.   Is this the first episode of spotting you have experienced?
         This question is important as the patient may have experienced spotting
         before and may have already miscarried and has ongoing bleeding.

b) What is your nursing diagnosis?
    Threatened Miscarriage

c) What triage category / score do you give this lady?
    ATS – 3 (30 minutes)
    CTAS – 3 (30 minutes)
    MTS – 3 (60 minutes)
    ESI – Level-2

Case Study Eight

a) What questions do you ask this mother?

I.   What was the mechanism of injury?

The reason for asking this question is the mechanism of injury will provide the triage nurse with information as to whether this could possibly be a fracture or a pulled elbow. If the child has fallen on her arm she may have sustained a fracture but if the mother tells you the child was about to fall over and she pulled her up by the wrist to stop her from falling she may have a pulled elbow. The two presentations are managed differently.

II.   Has the child had any pain relief?

This is important as the child will require pain relief if it is distressed it does not matter if the arm is fractured or a pulled elbow. The mother may have given the child pain relief prior to presentation and this is important to prevent double dosing.

III.   How much does the child weigh?

If the child has not had any pain relief this is important to calculate the dose of any pain relief required.

IV.   Has the child ever had a pulled elbow or fracture in this arm before?

This question will give the triage nurse an idea of any previous injuries sustained in the arm before.

b) What is your nursing diagnosis?
    Possible fracture in the fore arm / elbow
    Possible pulled elbow

c) What triage category / score do you give this child?
>ATS – 3 (30 minutes)
>CTAS – 3 (30 minutes) or 4 (60 minutes) depending on pain
>MTS – 3 (60 minutes)
>ESI – Level-4

Case Study Nine

a) What questions do you ask this young lady?

I. What is the mechanism of injury?

This question is important as it will give the triage nurse information as to how the injury occurred i.e. running, stationary; another player hit her knee, knocked off her feet. This question will allow the triage nurse to ascertain information that she can make a decision as to whether she thinks it could be a fracture or ligamentous in nature.

II. Did you walk on the injured leg straight away?

This gives information as to how painful and difficult the leg is to walk on, remembering the patient has walked into the ED with a moderate limp.

III. Have you taken any pain relief since the injury?

If the patient has not taken pain relief prior to presentation obtaining a pain score and providing pain relief is important prior to the medical staff examining the knee. The reason for this is the doctor / nurse practitioner may want to check the ligaments and this can be painful.

IV. Have you injured this knee before?

This may lead to previous injuries to this knee, the patient may have weak ligaments or they may have injured these ligaments in the past.

b) What is your nursing diagnosis?
>Possible ligamentous knee injury
>Possible soft tissue injury

c) What triage category / score do you give this lady?
>ATS – 4 (60 minutes)
>CTAS – 4 (60 minutes)
>MTS – 4 (120 minutes)
>ESI – Level-4

Case Study Ten

a) What questions do you ask?

    I.   When did the injury occur and what is the mechanism of injury?

        This is an important question as the type of injury suggests a fracture. It is important to know when the injury occurred as if there is a fracture it may have started healing already. The mechanism is important as this could possibly be a Boxer's fracture caused by punching something.

    II. Have you taken any pain relief?

        Again it is important to provide prompt pain relief and the correct type of pain relief for the injury. Also it is important to ascertain if the patient has medicated themselves prior to presentation to the ED.

    III. Is there any loss of sensation or numbness in the fingers or hand?

        This is an important question any loss of sensation may alter the decisions made by the triage nurse. It is important that the nurse assess the patient neurovascular status prior to assigning a triage priority / score.

b) What is your nursing diagnosis?

Fracture hand

Soft tissue injury to hand

c) What triage category / score do you give this man?

    ATS – 5 (120 minutes)

    CTAS – 4 (60 minutes)

    MTS – 3 (60 minutes)

    ESI – Level-4

Case Study Eleven

a) What questions do you ask?

    I.   When did you run out of your medication?

        The reason for asking is the patient may have taken her last tablet today or she may have run out a week ago. This is an important question as it leads on to the next question which will decide if the physician writes a new prescription or not.

II. Is there any chance you could be pregnant?

This is an important question as the patient should not be taking the Oral Contraceptive Pill (OCP) is there is a chance they could be pregnant the triage nurse should ask for a urine specimen and perform a pregnancy test. The physician may even ask for a pregnancy test done via a blood sample. The triage nurse may ask about unprotected sexual intercourse during the time the patient has not been taking the OCP.

b) What is your nursing diagnosis?

If the patient is not pregnant they require a prescription for the OCP.

If the patient is pregnant they may require some pregnancy counselling and support especially if they a young teenage woman.

c) What triage category / score do you give this young lady?

ATS – 5 (120 minutes)
CTAS – 5 (120 minutes)
MTS – 5 (240 minutes)
ESI – Level-4

Case Study Twelve

a) What questions do you ask this lady?

I. Where is the pain? What is the pain like?

The reason for asking this question is you are trying to find out if the patient is in labour. Asking the patient what the pain is like is important as she may describe it as the worst pain ever especially if the patient is having her first child. Also the nurse is trying to find out if the paint is coming and going like labour pains. The patient may describe pain that is coming and going either frequently or infrequently, this is important as it will impact the triage priority / level.

II. Have you experienced any vaginal loss?

The triage nurse is endeavouring to find out if the patient has experienced her waters breaking as this may indicate that she is in labour. The patient may have some vaginal bleeding this is important to ascertain also as this may effect not only the triage priority / level allocated but it can also affect the patient outcome.

III. Is this your first pregnancy? Has it been uneventful up until now?

This is an important question, if the patient is in labour it is vital to move quickly. She may have a lengthy labour being a first labour although if she is in labour the baby is very early and will require intervention from numerous interdisciplinary teams. If this has been an uneventful pregnancy this is important information.

IV. Have you experienced any abdominal pain before during this pregnancy?

The reason for asking this question is as the pregnancy progresses the abdomen stretches along with the ligaments in the abdomen that support the uterus, also some women can experience constipation. All of these reasons can be causes of abdominal pain. If the patient is not in labour then the cause of the abdominal pain may be something that can be treated simply and is not an emergency.

V. Do you have the pain now?

It is vital to ascertain if the patient has pain on presentation as the triage nurse may be able to call a colleague who can determine if the patient is in labour or not as this will affect the triage priority / level assigned to the patient.

b) What is your nursing diagnosis?

Abdominal pain cause by; constipation or stretching of the abdominal ligaments

Early labour

c) What triage category / score do you give this young lady?

ATS – 3 (30 minutes) / if labouring 2 (10 minutes)

CTAS – 3 (30 minutes) / if labouring contractions < 2 minutes 2 (10 minutes)

MTS – 3 (60 minutes) / if labouring 2 (10 minutes)

ESI – Level- 2

Case Study Thirteen

a) What questions do you ask this man?

I. What time did you fall?

This is an important question as it provides the nurse with a time line of the injury. The nurse is trying to ascertain when the patient fell and how long they have been in pain.

II. Where is the pain and does it move anywhere else?
The nurse will ask this question to localise where the pain is situated especially if they suspect the patient may have broken a rib. Radiation of the pain is also important to know as the patient may have other injuries.

III. Does it hurt to take a deep breath in?
The reason the nurse asks this question is they are looking for signs of a possible fractured rib or a pneumothorax. The answer the patient gives and the nurse's suspicions will affect the triage priority / level assigned to the patient. The nurse may even auscultate the patients chest and check for bilateral air entry, if there is decreased air entry on the left this may lead the nurse to suspect a pneumothorax.

IV. Do you have any other injuries? Did you hit your head?
The nurse is trying to determine if the patient sustained any other injuries during his fall, especially if he has a closed head injury. This is an important question for this age group as he may be at risk of a cerebral bleed.

V.   Are you on any medications?
This is an important question especially if the patient is taking a blood thinning medication such as aspirin, or warfarin. If the patient has fractured a rib or has a pneumothorax they are at risk of a haemo pneumothorax. This will affect the triage priority / level assigned the patient.

b) What is your nursing diagnosis?
Fractured rib
Pneumothorax
Haemo pneumothorax

c) What triage category / score do you give this man?
ATS – 3 (30 minutes) / 2 (10 minutes) if patient is unwell
CTAS – 3 (30 minutes)
MTS – 3 (60 minutes) / 2 (10 minutes) if unwell
ESI – Level- 3

It must be noted here that there is no right or wrong answer but a good patient outcome is important. If the nurse suspects the patient has the possibility of deterioration then it is better to up-triage the patient.

INDEX